Dr. Rabbit

By

ERIC B. HARE

Illustrations by *Siegfried Bohlmann*

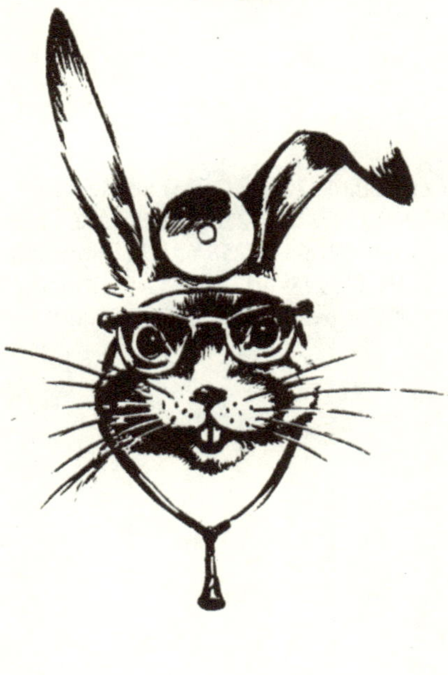

TEACH Services, Inc.
www.TEACHServices.com

PRINTED IN
THE UNITED STATES OF AMERICA

ISBN-13: 978-1-57258-278-1 (Paperback)
ISBN-13: 978-1-57258-651-2 (Hardback)
ISBN-13: 978-1-57258-652-9 (EBook)
Library of Congress Control Number: 2004104751

Published by
TEACH Services, Inc.
www.TEACHServices.com

Dedicated

To my junior friends all around the world who wrote such nice letters begging for more Dr. Rabbit stories, with the hope that all juniors everywhere will see that there is joy in serving Jesus, and that each one will find his own special place where he can serve God better than anyone else.

Contents

Dr. Rabbit Finds His Special Place 1

Jungle Graduation Exercises 13

Dr. Rabbit's First Baptisms 23

Dr. Rabbit Earns a New Degree 33

Dr. Bear Joins Up 44

The Curse of the Devil Tree 54

The Witch Doctor's Magic 64

Mamma Rabbit's Baby Patients 76

Triumphs and Defeats 85

A Real Doctor Comes 98

Good-by Dr. Rabbit and Mamma Rabbit 108

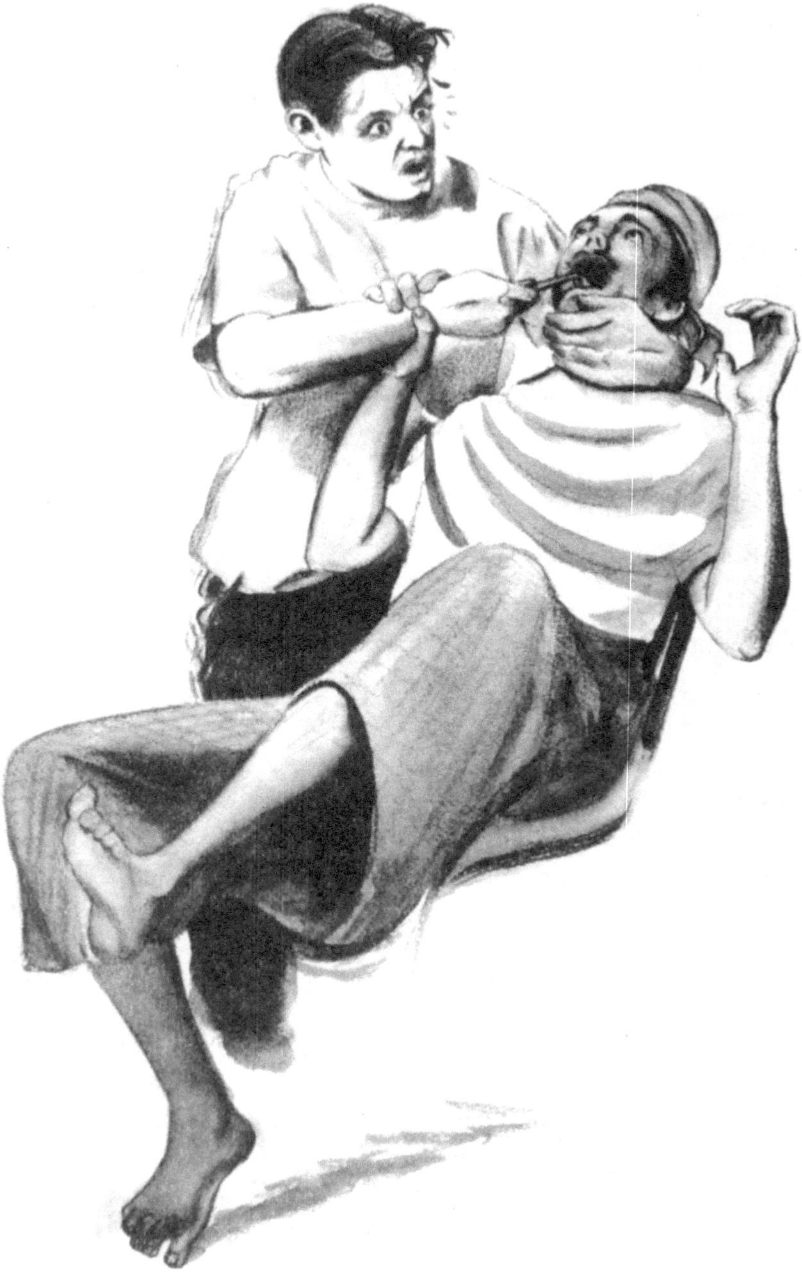

It was my first tooth, and by the time I fastened the forceps on the molar my knees were knocking together

Dr. Rabbit Finds His Special Place

ONCE upon a time, away down under in the country of Australia, there was born a little baby boy. His father was an Irishman, whose happy face radiated joy and gladness, and who taught his children to look for the cheerful side of life and to laugh. His mother was a very devoted American lady, and as soon as this little boy could talk she taught him to pray by repeating words phrase by phrase after her.

I was that little boy, and I can still remember part of that first prayer.

"And when I grow up . . .

"May I be a missionary . . .

"At the four corners of the earth . . .

"Preaching the gospel."

When I was big enough to say my own prayers I still prayed that prayer. When I was seven years old, at camp meeting Elder E. H. Gates told us children mission stories and showed us curios from the islands of the South Pacific. When I was eight years old Elder R. W. Munson told us stories from Singapore and taught us to sing "Jesus Loves Me" in the Malay language. I knew then that someday I *would*, I would be a missionary.

As I confided my heart's desire to my mother, she often used to say, "And remember, Eric, my son, Sister White says, 'Not more surely is the place prepared for us in the heavenly mansions than is the special place designated on earth where we are to work for God.'—*Christ's Object Lessons*, p. 327. So, somewhere, God has a special place for you, where you can serve Him better than anyone else."

"Where, Mother, where?" I used to whisper.

"Oh, somewhere," mother would answer. "And when you find that place, you'll know! You'll know it is the one God intended for you!"

I grew up and went to Avondale College, and when I graduated in 1913 I still prayed that prayer and was still looking for my special place. By this time I had fallen in love with a very sweet young lady—Agnes, one of the daughters of Elder J. E. Fulton, our pioneer missionary to Fiji. So naturally I decided to be a missionary in Fiji. That would be my special place.

"You'd better take the nurse's course, Eric," advised the brethren after my name had been discussed on the committee. "We are recommending that all our island missionaries take the nurse's course, not only for the work's sake but also for their own sake. You can never tell; maybe you will be stationed many miles from a doctor or a hospital."

"That's right, Eric," added Captain Jones. "A few of us are trail blazers, but we need medical missionaries to establish the work that we open up."

I loved and respected the brethren, but I idolized dear old courageous Captain Jones. During my college years I had often seen him and heard him, and in my heart of hearts, being a missionary meant being a missionary just like him. So I wholeheartedly took a two-year nurse's course given to men in the Sydney Sanitarium at that time.

By March of 1915, with only six more months of my nurse's course to go, I was making good progress learning Fijian in my spare time, with Agnes, my own ladylove, as my teacher, when Elder A. G. Daniells came to Australia on his way around the world to study how to reorganize the work of the church. I was thrilled when Elder Fulton introduced me to him. "This is my soon-to-be son-in-law," said Elder Fulton.

''I'm glad to know you," said Elder Daniells, and I felt his eyes looking right through me. "You are Pastor Robert Hare's son?"

"Yes," I nodded.

"Nearly finished your nurse's course?"

"Yes," I nodded again.

He was too great a man, and I was too unimportant a young fellow to say more, but those few words gave me a great lift. Maybe Elder Daniells would put a word in for me and help me to become the missionary I wanted to be.

He certainly did help. But I had no idea how soon his help would come, nor how earth shaking that help would be when it did come.

From Australia Elder Daniells went on to India, and in just a few weeks we heard from him. He sent a cablegram to Elder Fulton:

"We need a young medical missionary for a new mission station among the Karen spirit worshipers of Burma. Will Eric and Agnes accept the invitation?"

"Burma?" I gasped.

"What about Fiji?" added Agnes, equally nonplused.

"Where's Burma anyway?"

"Maybe we should take time to pray and make sure God really needs us in Burma."

We were all quiet and speechless for a moment, then I replied slowly, "I don't need to pray anymore about it. I've prayed all my life to be a missionary, at the four corners of the earth. And I believe God speaks through His ministers. I just felt something was going to happen, the way Elder Daniells looked at me, and I am ready to go to Burma if the Lord wants me there. What about you, Agnes?"

There were tears in her eyes as she replied calmly, "Whither thou goest, I will go."

So we were married in June. I graduated from the nurse's course in September, and in October 1915, we sailed away to Burma, the land of the golden pagodas and Karen spirit worshipers.

Pastor George Hamilton, the Karen Mission superintendent, and Mary Gibbs, the dispensary nurse, met us at the Rangoon wharf and entertained us with hair-raising stories of God's providence in helping to procure the land for the new Karen mission at Kamamaung, on the banks of the great Salween River. They were already living there in temporary houses while the mission house and the dispensary were being built. Nurse Mary Gibbs already had her hands full looking after sick ones in the shade of the mango trees. She could speak the Karen language, and it would have been wonderful if she could have stayed on right there. But she had so much experience that it was planned for her to head up a new school for girls as soon as possible. This is why we had been called to be the medical assistants at this new station.

"First, you will be given six months free for language study," said Pastor Hamilton. "Then you will roll up your sleeves and start right in with us. The dispensary will be built by that time, and also a bamboo house for you."

That night when we were alone I looked at my wife and she looked at me, and our eyes were full of question marks. Would this be it—our own special place? Would it?

In six months we could read our Karen Bibles somewhat haltingly and speak Karen a little hesitantly, so it was time to go to work. We traveled by river steamer and motor launch to our mission station. We moved into our little bamboo-and-leaf house, so kindly prepared by Pastor Hamilton, and with my sleeves rolled up I reported to Nurse Mary Gibbs at the dispensary for duty the next morning.

Nurse Gibbs smiled a big welcome and pointed to a white doctor's coat hanging on the door. I put it on and looked about. There were perhaps twenty people sitting around on the veranda and on the steps, waiting for their turn to be treated or proudly showing off their bandages and describing the treatment they had already received from the white woman doctor. Some had sore eyes, some had ringworm, some had fever, some had ugly tropical ulcers, and most of the children had worms or stomachache.

"Here's a man who needs to have a tooth pulled out, Doctor," said Nurse Gibbs pleasantly. "How about your doing it for him?"

Me? Pull a tooth? Doctor? Of course, I was certainly not a doctor. I had only a nurse's diploma. However, I realized that the Karen word for doctor was used for all professional people, and I could have felt very important, except that I suddenly realized that my nurse's course did not include any dentistry. I began to whisper, "But, Nurse Gibbs, I've never pulled a tooth in all my—"

Nurse Gibbs was merciless. "Here are the forceps, the oil of cloves, and the lance and elevator if you need them." She placed a small tray in my hands. "And there is your patient!"

There was no way out. After all, was not this what I had come to Burma to do? All right, then, I would do it. I asked the patient to open his mouth and show me the tooth. Fortunately, it was a first molar, easy to get at, and it was very loose. I picked up a small swab and dipped it in the oil of cloves. I noticed that my hand was trembling. That would never do. Me, a strong young man, trembling! I painted around the tooth with the oil of cloves and said to myself, "Mr. Hare, control yourself! Control yourself!" But it did no good. The trembling extended to my arms. I picked up the forceps, and by the time I had fastened them on the tooth my knees were knocking together. I broke out with cold perspiration all over, then suddenly the tooth was out! I'm not quite sure yet whether I pulled that tooth or whether it just fell out with the trembling.

"Well, Doctor, you lived through that." Nurse Gibbs smiled knowingly. "Now see what that old man who has been sitting over there so patiently wants."

I went over and sat beside the old gentleman and inquired kindly, "What can I do for you?"

"I need some medicine for my eye," he said.

"Does it hurt?"

"No, not much, but I can't see out of it."

One glance told me that he had a cataract in his eye. I opened my mouth to explain that he would have to go to the government hospital for that, but he hastened to explain how it happened.

"You see, two years ago I had fever; my head was hot but my feet were cold. Then one day the cold wind in my feet began to work its way up my legs. Do you see?" He stood up suddenly to demonstrate the movement of the cold wind. "Well, at last the cold wind came to the hot wind in my stomach. There was a terrible noise. I thought I would surely die. But the cold wind kept coming up and up, through my neck, over my head, and it settled in my right eye. From that time on, it has just gotten worse, till now I can't see out of that eye at all."

I nodded my head to show I understood him, and tried not to smile.

"And so," he went on, "I wish you could give me some wind medicine that would drive that cold wind down through my body and out of my feet again. They say you have all kinds of wind medicine here." He was so serious. It was no smiling matter to him.

"I will write you a letter to give to the doctor in the Moulmein Government Hospital," I said. "He can operate and you will be able to see again. We do not have the instruments or the experience to take out that kind of cold wind here in our dispensary."

He looked so disappointed. Go to Moulmein? Why, he had never traveled that far in all his life. And where could he find money for such a trip? He searched my face to make sure I was telling him the truth, then slowly he turned away and went back to his jungle home again, hoping that maybe, someday, somewhere, he could find some magic wind medicine for his eye.

"Poor old fellow!" I reported to Nurse Gibbs. "He doesn't know how much he made my heart ache. How I wish I could have been a real doctor. How it hurt to have to tell him there is nothing I can do and to send him away disappointed."

"To be sure," agreed Nurse Gibbs, "your heart will often ache. But you will find that we nurses *can* care for at least ninety per cent of the needs of these dear jungle people, and the simple thanks and appreciation of those you can help will make your life here very rewarding."

For the next few weeks I learned to appreciate Nurse Gibbs more than words can ever express. In addition to her six years of mission experience, she had been privileged to take a special course in tropical diseases. Every day I discovered things my nurse's diploma had not prepared me for, and it was she who taught me how to diagnose and treat the various jungle fevers such as malaria, dengue, and relapsing fever. It was she who taught me how to lance boils and sew up wounds and care for jungle accidents. And it was she who taught me how to mix our famous God-worshiper's medicines.

One morning as I reported for duty, Nurse Gibbs said, "You're a pretty good dentist by this time, Doctor. See what you can do for that little two-year-old crying over there in its mother's arms."

I slipped into my white coat, washed my hands, and went quickly to the crying baby.

"Doctor, I think my baby has the toothache," said the worried mother.

After a difficult moment I at last succeeded in opening the baby's mouth and looking inside. To be sure, there were signs of infection. In fact, one tooth had rotted right out. I gently cleaned up the place where the tooth had been. There was still something white at the bottom of the sore. It could be a root to a baby tooth! I selected a pointed pair of forceps and tried to see if I could pull that white thing out. I pulled three white things out, but they were not pieces of tooth. They were three wiggling maggots!

"Oh, thank you, Doctor," cried the happy mother. "Thank you so much." The baby was fast asleep, almost, before I started on the next patient.

As our patients increased in numbers, Agnes was pressed into the baby-care department, and she was soon quite expert in washing and bathing them, binding up their sores, and administering the much-depended-on castor oil.

One day after the morning rush was over, Nurse Gibbs went back to her room to work on the translation of a book, *The Christian Sabbath*, leaving me in charge of the dispensary. I was chatting with the several patients who still sat around when a man came rushing up the front steps calling out, "Doctor! Doctor! Come quick! A man has been stung!"

"Where is he?" I asked.

"Three miles away in Wakawkyi," he replied breathlessly. "Come quick!"

"All right," I replied. "I'll come with you right away."

"It sounds pretty bad," I said to myself as I opened up my medicine bag. "Now, what is good for stings?" Ammonia is very good for stings, so I put a bottle of ammonia into the bag. Then I remembered that when I was a little boy my mother used to rub the bluing bag over my bee stings, so I ran over to the house and got the bluing bag from Agnes. Then I remembered that someone had told me that onion juice was good, too, so I put an onion into my bag. Then away we went through the jungle to see the man who had been stung. Can you imagine my horror when I arrived at a little bamboo house and found a man lying on the floor with his right arm nearly torn off at the shoulder. “Why didn’t you tell me the truth?” I said to the man who had called me. “This man hasn’t been stung; he has been almost murdered!”

“Oh, no, doctor, he hasn’t been murdered. He’s been stung.”

“Whatever in the world could sting a man like that?” I asked a little indignantly. “Why,” he said, “an elephant!”

My mouth opened wide. My eyes bugged out. I felt wheels going around in my head as I realized that my limited knowledge of the Karen language had limited stings to bees or wasps. Whereas, in reality, these people have only one word for *sticking*, and whether you are stuck by a bee or a pin or an elephant’s tusk, you are stung just the same. Fortunately, there were other things besides onions and bluing bags that we always carried in the medicine bag, and before long the wound was carefully washed and sewn up and bandaged. Then with his arm supported in a sling, the patient sat up. Wriggling the fingers of the injured arm, he grinned and said, “Thank you, Doctor. Thank you!” Then reaching out his good hand, he took hold of mine and squeezed it lovingly.

My heart was full of happiness and my feet were light as feathers as I raced home to report about my “stung” patient to Nurse Gibbs. There was a grin of approval on her face as she replied, “You’ll be a great jungle doctor someday.” She paused a moment. The grin on her face broadened till it spread from ear to ear, then she said, “Do you know what?”

I said, “What?”

She said, “The people keep asking your name, and I tell them ‘Hare.’ But that has no meaning for them. Then I try to give them the meaning in Karen, but their language makes no difference between Hare and Rabbit. Then their eyes brighten up and they nod their heads with seeming approval, and they say 'Thara Pa-Deh! Thara Pa-Deh!' which means 'Dr. Rabbit, Dr. Rabbit.' So don't be surprised if you find them calling you Dr. Rabbit someday."

That evening in our little leaf-and-bamboo house I said to Agnes, "I like these people!"

And she said, "I do too."

"You can't imagine how I felt when that man said Thank you and squeezed my hand."

"I can too," replied Agnes. "I feel the same way when I put the babies I've been treating back into their mothers' arms."

"Fancy them calling me Dr. Rabbit! I wonder what it is that makes them like that name?"

"Someday we will find out," Agnes said. "And I suppose they will call me Mamma Rabbit." She grinned.

"Do you know what?" I whispered.

"What?" Agnes whispered back.

"This is beginning to feel like our own special place."

Agnes sighed and smiled a very satisfied smile and whispered, "I feel it is too."

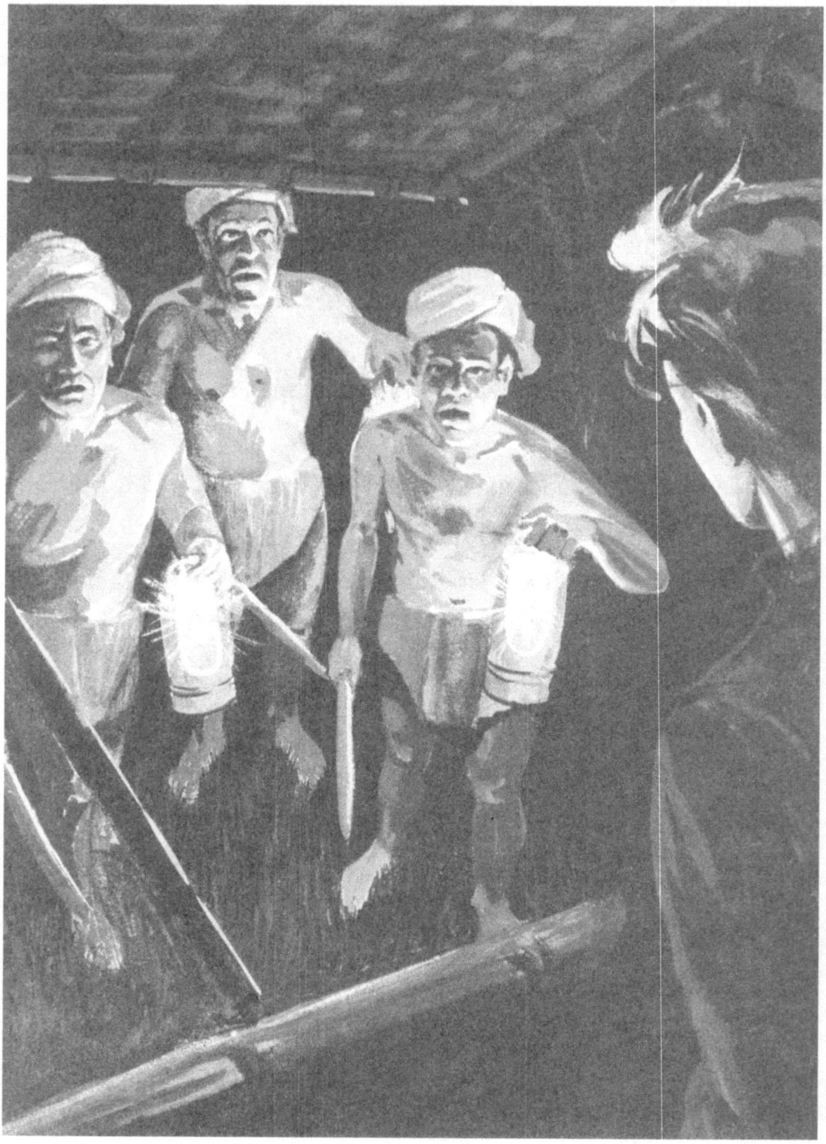

I saw three almost-naked men, each holding a sword-like knife in one hand and a small oil lamp in the other.

Jungle Graduation Exercises

DOCTOR! Doctor! Letter! Letter! Doctor!"

It was about midnight, and I was sleeping alone in our little leaf-and-bamboo house. Agnes and Nurse Gibbs had run down to Rangoon for a day or two to do some shopping. The Hamiltons were in the mission bungalow some five hundred yards away. I was a young man. I worked hard, long hours, and slept like a log. Therefore it took a moment or two for the cry, "Doctor! Doctor!" to reach my brain. When it did, it took another moment or two for my sound-asleep body to respond. But at last I managed to throw back the covers and step out of bed. However, that was as far as I could get, and that was all I could do, for looking out of the propped-open bamboo window to the ground six feet below, there I saw three almost-naked men. Their bodies were greased. Each held a gleaming sword-like knife in his right hand and a small oil lamp in his left.

My eyes opened wide, my hair stood on end, my ears swelled out, and I stood there petrified. How long I stood there motionless I cannot tell, but little by little I became conscious that they were handing up to me a piece of paper and saying, "Letter! Letter! Doctor! Doctor!" Little by little, encouraged by the fact that the men made no movement to indicate they had come to chop me up, I swallowed hard, stroked my hair down, patted my ears back into position, then reached out and took the letter. Quickly I lighted my lamp and read:

"Dear Mr. Hare:

"An Indian marijuana addict has run amok here in Kamamaung, and has chopped up a Burmese woman and her twelve-year-old son. Bring all your needles and sutures and see what you can do.

BALDWIN

"*Tennasserim District Forest Officer.*"

Suddenly I was very much awake. I had met most of the government officers as they traveled up and down the district and stayed in the government rest house just one mile south of our mission, and I knew Mr. Baldwin.

I tried getting more information from the greased-up messengers, but that was useless. They were Burmese and I couldn't understand their language, neither could they understand my Karen. However, I sprang into action. I was clothed in seconds, and in a few minutes I had loaded all the needles and sutures I had into my medicine bag, and off we went. We walked single file, two of the greased messengers going ahead, and one following after me. I soon figured out that they had greased their bodies in case they came to grips with the crazed addict, who had disappeared after his brutal attack, and now might be anywhere. The men jumped at every crackling sound, and held their knives at the ready. I jumped too. Those crackling sounds could also be tigers, for this was tiger country. Fortunately, we saw neither the maniac nor a tiger, and in twenty minutes we rounded a curve in the jungle path and entered the village.

The street was ablaze with a dozen bonfires. The villagers, pale-faced and fearful, stood around peering into the shadows.

"The doctor has come!" shouted those nearest, and the cry was taken up, all through the village. From the groups near the first fire stepped the headman. He spoke Karen. "Oh, I'm so glad you've come," he said. "It's terrible! I don't know if they are still alive or not." As he led me toward the house where they were, he gave me the gruesome particulars. We reached the house. He opened the door, and pushed me in. "I can't bear to look at them," he said as he closed the door on me.

With the light of my lantern I saw two bodies. The mother lay on her cotton mattress on the floor. The boy was on his mattress on the other side of the room. And there was a lot of blood. It was the first time I had seen so much human blood. It had a strange heavy sweet nauseating smell. Suddenly the boy began to yell and shout.

"Oh, ho!" I said to myself. "He is still alive anyway, so I'll look after him first." I stepped over his mother's body. She was motionless. "Most likely dead," I said to myself. As my foot stepped onto her mattress the blood oozed out around my shoe, and as it did I felt my head begin to swim. Around and around it went. I realized that I was about to faint. I had to do something. I couldn't just fall down there in the middle of this mess. So I talked out loud, and severely to myself, "No, you don't, Dr. Rabbit. This is no time or place to faint! Keep your wits about you!"

It worked! In a few seconds I was kneeling by the frightened boy doing my best to comfort him. There was a horrible gash in his neck, but neither the jugular vein nor the artery had been severed. Two fingers of one hand had been cut right through the bones, but in a very few minutes I had a bandage on his neck and a splint on his fingers. I took him to the door and handed him to the headman. "Please go and call Mr. Baldwin," I said. "Tell him I need his help."

In a very quick minute Mr. Baldwin opened the door. He took one look and began to say, "I say, Hare—say—you've got—" His voice faltered. I looked up. His face was as white as a sheet. I realized he was going to faint and if he did he would fall right into the middle of everything. I sprang to his help and succeeded in catching him as he fell limp into my arms.

I said to the headman, "Put some cold water on his face, and have the men carry him back to the rest house." Then addressing the crowd I said, "I need help. Isn't there anyone who will come and help me?" For what seemed like a very long moment no one moved. Then a little old grandma who spoke Karen volunteered.

"I'll come and help you, Doctor," she said. "I'll come. I'm so old and skinny the evil spirits couldn't do anything to me anyway."

We knelt one on each side of the apparently dead woman. Her forehead was split right open till I could see the tissue under the skull bone. Her left cheek was sliced almost off, just hanging by the flesh of the lower jaw, and through the hole I could see her teeth and tongue. The flesh of her right arm had been opened up to the bone on two sides of the humerus bone. Her left arm had been hacked right off below the elbow! I looked at my little old lady helper. But nothing upset her. She was game. She knew exactly how to help—holding, tying, pinning up the bandages. We could feel no pulse in the right arm. We could detect no heartbeat. But from the severed forearm the bleeding still came in feeble jerks. "Maybe she is still alive," I whispered.

"Ugh! Maybe," grunted my helper.

First we put a tourniquet on the severed arm and stopped the bleeding. Then we carefully bound up the split forehead, and then we bound the almost severed cheek into position. Last, we bound the flesh of the upper right arm into position.

"Get me some hot milk," I whispered.

In a few minutes it was brought. I put a teaspoonful to the lips of the apparently dead woman, and she swallowed it! I gave her another—and another—and another. She swallowed half a cup of warm milk, then she opened her eyes and looked at me! Another spoonful or two and then she spoke! ''I'm not going to die," she said slowly and painfully.

At once I went into conference with the headman. "Look here," I said. "I don't have enough sutures to sew her up. I've just been able to give her first aid."

"The nearest government hospital is sixty miles down the river," said the headman hopelessly. "It's a police case," I said. "I think you ought to send her there anyway."

"Do you think she can live that long?"

"I think it is a miracle she has lived this long. She must have been attacked more than an hour ago!"

"More like two hours!"

"Well, she is alive now. Let us get things moving," I urged.

The headman did get things moving. He had some men make a bamboo litter, and we placed the patient on it. He commandeered the largest canoe in the village and selected six of the strongest men to paddle it downstream. I wrote a letter to the doctor at the Paan Government Hospital, and at 2:30 A.M. I pushed them off and wished them a good trip. As the canoe bearing the unfortunate woman sped off and slowly disappeared in the darkness, I stood there for a moment alone with my thoughts. Then suddenly there was the sound of running, and a voice coming toward me called, “Doctor, Doctor, do you want this?”

It was too dark to see what the man was bringing me, but I put out my hands anyway to receive what he had for me. Into my hands he placed the cold dead arm that had been hacked off! “No! No!” I gasped. “We can’t do anything with that anymore. Take it away and bury it.”

Slowly I turned and made my way to Mr. Baldwin in the government rest house. He was wide-eyed and pale. “Sit down, Mr. Hare,” he said, “and tell me all about it.”

So I did. I sat down and told him about the poor woman, and how badly she was cut up. I told him about the game little old lady who helped me put the bandages on. I told him I felt as if a corpse had opened its eyes and spoken to me, and ended with the dead arm being placed in my hands.

Mr. Baldwin shuddered. “I don’t see how you can do it!” he said.

Then I was quiet for a few moments, for I didn’t want to tell him how near I had come to keeling over and fainting myself. But I can tell you now. That was my graduation! After that I was a real jungle doctor. No amount of blood, no degree of being burned or mauled by tigers or gored by buffaloes or elephants, ever made my head go round and round or my heart feel like fainting anymore.

Mr. Baldwin and I talked for two or three hours exchanging stories of devil trees and devil doctors, evil spirits and ghosts, and such things that are common experiences of the people in the jungle villages. At last the dawn broke, and I took my way back to my leaf-and-bamboo house. After washing up and shaving I ran over to the Hamiltons and told them of the exciting graduation exercises for Dr. Rabbit.

In a few days Agnes and Nurse Gibbs returned from the city. They both smiled their approval of my act of midnight mercy. By this time I also had the news that the man who had run amok had been caught and was in jail, and that the poor woman reached the government hospital still alive and had been sewn up, but her life was hanging in the balance. So also was the addict's life hanging in the balance, for if the woman died, he would be hanged, and if she lived he would be given a life sentence in the Adaman Island penitentiary. Then, because the days were so full of so many other interesting cases, we just forgot about this attempted murder case.

Six weeks went by. One morning while I was busy treating patients with sore eyes, ringworm, and fever, up the stairs into the dispensary came a woman with her face all scarred like a crazy patchwork quilt. The scars didn't look like smallpox scars or tiger-claw scars. I looked at her with a puzzled expression on my face till she said, "Doctor, don't you remember me?"

I replied, "No, Auntie. I can't remember ever seeing anyone with such strange-looking scars on her face."

Then with a deft movement she threw her shawl from her left arm, revealing a stump where once her arm had been hacked off. "Well, now do you know me?" she cried as tears welled up in her eyes.

Yes, then I remembered. I couldn't talk for a moment as the memories of that midnight nightmare rushed into my mind. And while I stood there, before I could stop her, she fell to her knees at my feet, and putting her one good arm around them she sobbed out her thanks. "Oh, if you hadn't come that night when the marijuana fiend ran amok and cut me up, I surely would have died. But you weren't afraid of the night. You weren't afraid of the tigers. You came, and now my son and I both live."

"Aye! Aye!" chorused the other patients who had gathered around. "Of course he came! Of course you live! Isn't his name Dr. Rabbit?" said an old man.

Everyone laughed. I did too, and wondered what was coming next. "Didn't the rabbit save the elephant's life when the tiger was going to eat him all up?"

"Aye! Aye!" chorused the group.

"And didn't the rabbit tell the horse how to get two sets of teeth so he could whinny?" went on the old one.

"Aye! Aye!" chorused the group.

"And didn't grandfather rabbit overcome grandfather alligator, and pull his tongue out and plant it on the tall tree?"

"Aye! Aye!" chorused the group louder than ever.

"And didn't the rabbit frighten the tiger so that he ran away with the monkey tied on his back, and the jungle bushes were so thick that the monkey's head and arms kept catching in the branches and his stomach was stretched so much that to this day it is the thinnest part of his body?"

"Aye! Aye!"

"And wasn't the rabbit the best lawyer? And didn't he always win his cases?"

"Aye! Aye!"

"And wasn't the rabbit the best doctor? And didn't his medicine cure every disease?"

"Aye! Aye!"

Suddenly I realized that the old man was referring to their animal folklore tales. I had read some of them already in my study of the Karen language, and had noticed with some satisfaction that the rabbit was believed to have very superior talents. Still I was hardly prepared for what he said next.

"Well then, isn't this white doctor *our* Dr. Rabbit?"

"Aye! Aye!"

"And won't he overcome all our sickness enemies?"

"Aye! Aye!"

"And won't we all get better if we eat his medicine?"

"Aye! Aye! " chorused the group, and smiling to each other they said, "Sure! He's *our* Dr. Rabbit. He's our Dr. Rabbit."

That evening in our little bamboo-and-leaf home, I said to Agnes, "I sure do like these people!"

She said, "I do too."

And I said, "You know, I feel I belong right here."

And she said, "I do too."

"Funny, isn't it, they're calling me their Dr. Rabbit."

"Yes, and they are calling me their Mamma Rabbit too! Funny, isn't it?" Agnes sighed a happy sigh.

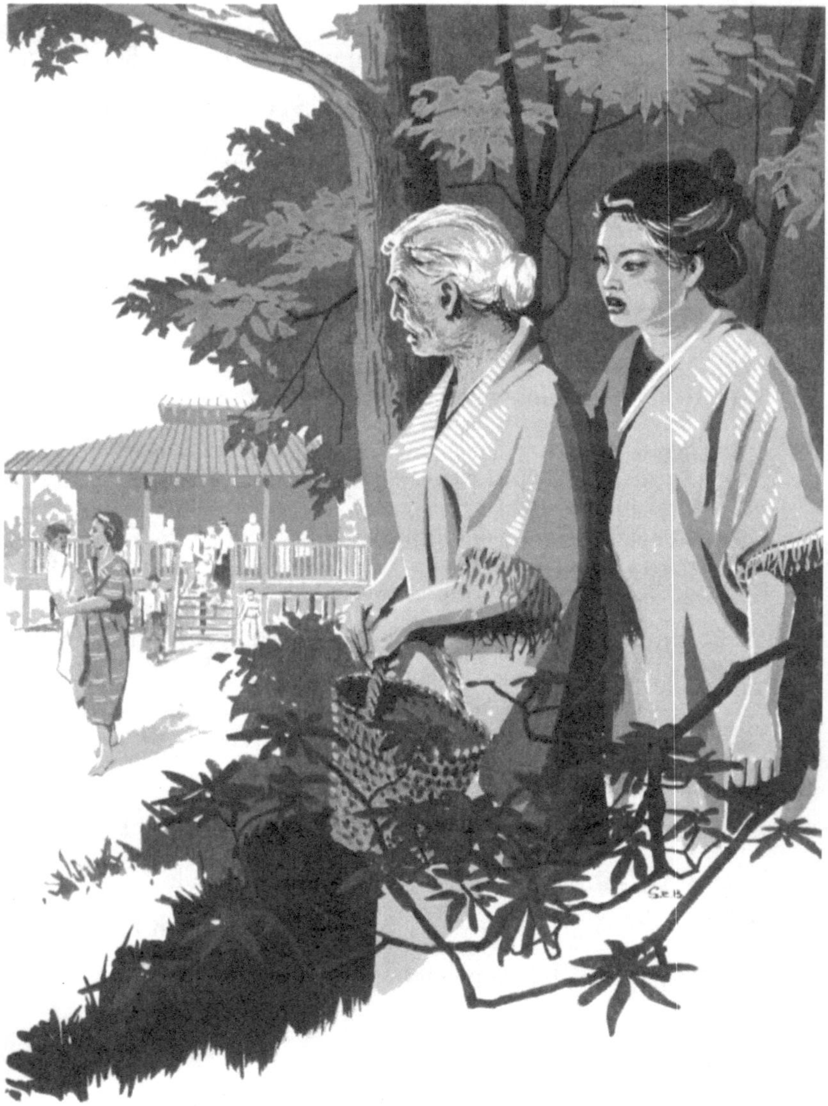

"Wait," whispered Rippling Water to Fair One. "Let us watch and see if the white ones really do eat babies."

Dr. Rabbit's First Baptisms

"DID y' hear? Did y' hear? Did y' hear?" called old Rippling Water excitedly as she gathered some old ladies around her in the village of Kawmalay, eight miles from our mission. "The God worshipers have built a sickness house on the bank of the big river, among the coconut palms. And they say there is a white lady doctor there, and a white man doctor whom they call their Dr. Rabbit, and I'm going down to see them, I am, I am."

"Dr. Rabbit?" gasped the excited women. "Did you say his name is Dr. Rabbit?"

"Yes, and they say their medicine is powerful, and everybody who eats their medicine gets better. I'm going down to see them, I am, I am."

"White people? God worshipers?" hissed some unbelieving ones. "White *dawtakas*! That's what they are. Their fathers are evil spirits and their mothers are ghosts! That's what they are, they're *dawtakas*! Of course their medicine is powerful. Once you eat their medicine you come under their power, and then they will eat you, and your babies too."

"Ha! Ha! Ha!" laughed the crowd.

"I don't care what you say," said old Rippling Water defiantly. "I am going down to see them, I am, I am." "You'd better be careful! You'd better be careful!" said the old ladies solemnly. "You know the devils don't like us to have anything to do with the God worshipers, and if you do go down, and then any trouble comes to our village, it will all be your fault. And if the devils get angry, it will be your fault, and we won't let you live here anymore. We won't! We won't!"

"I don't care what you say or what you do," insisted Rippling Water. "I am going down to see them, I am." And she did. The very next day, calling her eighteen year-old daughter, Fair One, to accompany her, down to the dispensary she came. Through the rice fields and the bamboo forests they walked without a care. Arriving at the great Salween River, they were fortunate to find a fisherman friend who willingly ferried them across in his canoe. Then as they came within view of the sickness house, their hearts began to palpitate and their knees began to tremble. "You'd better be careful. You'd better be careful!" the old ladies had said.

"Wait," whispered Rippling Water to Fair One. "Let us wait here in the bushes and watch awhile. After all, they said the white ones were *dawtakas* and that they ate babies. There is no harm in waiting awhile to see if it is true." So they waited behind some bushes where they could see the dispensary and the people as they came and went. While they waited, a mother went in with a crying babe in her arms. A man went in groaning in pain as he held an abscessed hand. Soon the mother came out with a happy, smiling baby in her arms. Then the man came out with a clean bandage on his hand, his face wreathed in happiness.

Rippling Water gasped. Catching Fair One by the arm, she said,

"Come, what are we waiting for? They are not *dawtakas*. They don't eat babies. Look! The babies go in crying; they come out laughing. They go in sick; they come out well. They go in dead and they come out alive! Come on. Let us go."

Through the gate, up the steps, and into the dispensary they came. For a moment they stood petrified at all they saw. There was the white lady doctor washing a man's sore hand. She was so gentle. She put some ointment on it, then she put a clean bandage around it and said with a smile, "There you are, Uncle. That feels better, doesn't it? Come again tomorrow and I'll give it another treatment."

Old Rippling Water couldn't believe her ears. "The white woman speaks our words! She speaks our words!"

Nurse Gibbs looked up and smiled. "Of course we do, Auntie," she said. "How I wish I could come and visit you in your village homes. Then you'd know. But there are so many sick people and so many sick babies coming all day long, that I never get a chance to go visiting. Do you know what I need, Auntie?" Nurse Gibbs turned to another patient while she talked. "I need a girl about eighteen years old to help me wash bandages and learn how to give babies their castor oil, and how to put eye drops in sore eyes."

Rippling Water's heart began to pound. She looked at *her* girl, Fair One. Nurse Gibbs hadn't noticed her yet. The lady doctor was speaking again. "Auntie, do you know a girl who would like to come and live with me?"

For just a second Rippling Water and Fair One looked at each other. Then pulling her forward, Rippling Water said, "Would my Fair One do?"

Nurse Gibbs looked at Fair One and was thrilled. “Would you—would she—like to come?” “Of course she would like to come. There are many things she can do to help the lady doctor.” Rippling Water was grinning happily.

So it was that Fair One came to live at the mission and became the first national assistant at the Karen dispensary. Her coming made all on the mission happy. But away back in the village where Rippling Water lived the old ladies whispered to one another, “Did y’ hear? Did y’ hear? That woman has let her daughter go to live with the God worshipers. Now, you’ll see; it won’t be long before they eat her all up. It won’t! It won’t!”

Of course, the God worshipers didn’t eat Fair One. They taught her how to work, and with her fearless help and continued presence, the dispensary work increased and prospered.

About a year after this, our staff was increased by a young Karen graduate from our Meiktila Training School, Thara Peter by name, and with his help we soon had a small but very much alive mission school established. The future began to look bright. Then suddenly Nurse Gibbs went home on furlough, and Pastor and Mrs. Hamilton were called to care for the English-speaking church in Rangoon. This left Dr. Rabbit and Mamma Rabbit in charge of the whole mission, with Thara Peter and Fair One, to run everything—school, dispensary, and all. But we were not alone. The God who had called us was with us. Soon we began to see fruits for our labors.

I can never forget the day when Fair One said to me, “Look, Dr. Rabbit, I’ve been here more than two years now. I’ve learned to work and I’ve learned to read. Every day I read part of the Golden Book. In that Book I've found Jesus, and I believe He is the Son of God. Doctor, I would like to be baptized and become a God worshiper *too*."

I was almost too happy for words. At last I managed to say, ''I'm so glad, Fair One. Next time your mother comes down we will ask her what she thinks of it."

In a few days Rippling Water came down, and as soon as we told her about Fair One's desire she replied, "Well, I don't mind if she does become a God worshiper. We have worshiped the devils and the evil spirits all our lives, and they are no good. And, Doctor, I'll tell you what. Maybe, when I know a little more, I might become a God worshiper too."

We sent to Rangoon for an ordained minister to come and perform the baptism, and whom do you think they sent? Pastor A. H. Williams, who had been with Pastor Hamilton when the location for the mission was selected. What a happy day it was for us! Our little mission family of workers and school children stood on the riverbank singing "Happy day, happy day, When Jesus washed my sins away," while Fair One was baptized. But away back in the village where Rippling Water lived it was a different story. "Did y' hear? Did y' hear?" cried the old ladies in anger. "Those God worshipers took that woman's daughter and dipped her right down underneath the water! Now they'll come to our village and catch all of us and dip us all down under the water. Oh, what will we do? What will we do?"

"We won't let old Rippling Water live here any longer! We won't!" shouted one.

"No, we won't! We won't!" chorused the rest of the angry ones. So they called the Buddhist priest and had him curse poor old Rippling

Water, her house, and her children. With sticks and stones they drove her away.

"Doctor, Doctor, what shall I do now?" she pleaded, as she told us the sad story the next day.

"I think their anger will cool down soon," I said. "You see, Rippling Water, the British Government guarantees religious freedom to each of its subjects. So why don't you just visit around with some of your friends and relatives for a week or two." She followed my suggestion, and all was well for a little while.

But back in her village all was not well. You see, there was no one left to take care of the empty house that had been cursed. So there was no one there to put a handful of rice on the spirit altar and to ring the spirit gong each morning. This made the evil spirits angry, so they said, and the evil spirits came down and haunted that house. At night the village folk were terrified with the screaming and yelling and groaning that issued forth from that cursed empty house.

"We can't stand it," said the old men as they gathered in the village council. "The haunted house is worse than the old woman. It is! It is! It is!"

"Then what shall we do?" asked the headman.

"I know. I know," said one. "Let us burn it down."

"Fine! Fine!" chorused the old men.

"Then *you* strike the first match," ordered the headman.

"Oh, no, not me," said the man who had suggested the idea. "I'm afraid of the devils. Let someone else start the fire."

"Not me!"

"Not me!"

"Not me!" said everyone. Not one of them was brave enough to strike the first match to burn the house down. "I know! I know!" cried another. "Let us pull it down! You pull a board, I'll pull a board, everyone of us will pull a board. The devils can't kill all of us!"

"Fine! Fine!" chorused the old men. "Then *you* pull the first board off," ordered the headman.

"Oh, no, no, not me!" said the one who had suggested the idea. "I'm afraid."

"So am I."

"So am I."

"So am I," said they all. Not one of them was brave enough to pull the first board off the haunted house.

"I know! I know!" at last said another. "Let us send for the old woman and make her come and pull it down herself."

"Fine! Fine!" chorused the old men. "Then *you* go and call the old woman," ordered the headman. "All right. All right. I'll go," the man agreed, and off he went.

The very next day poor old Rippling Water stood weeping before me. "How can I pull a house down?" she cried. "I'm only a little old woman. How I wish I could sell the old house. I'd be glad to go and live somewhere else."

Now, strange as it may seem, just five days before this I had received two hundred rupees—it was part of a Thirteenth Sabbath Offering overflow—with which to build a new boys' house for our growing school. As I stood looking at poor old Rippling Water in tears, a bright idea came to me. "Are the posts of your house still good?" I asked.

"Just as good as the day the house was built," she replied. "We got the best hardwood posts."

"Are the floor boards still good?" "Just as good as can be."

"Then will you let *me* buy your house?" I said. "I'll go over with some of our big boys and we'll pull it down."

"Oh, Doctor, if you could do that I'd sell it to you for fifty rupees."

The next day we went together to the village council. I said, "Gentlemen, would you be willing for me to pay Rippling Water fifty rupees for the posts and the floor boards of her old house? Then I'd come with some of my big boys and *we* could pull it down and cart it away."

"Fine! Fine!" they chorused. They didn't care what the devils did to the God worshipers—the worse the better, the quicker, the better. So the headman said, "Come tomorrow."

"It will take me three or four days to get ready," I said. "Then I'll come."

In a few days Thara Peter and I with a dozen of our big boys arrived with half a dozen bullock wagons and several crowbars and hammers, ready for business.

"They've come! They've come!" shouted the villagers excitedly. "Come and see what the devils will do to them."

They stood around in a big circle, fully expecting the devils to pounce upon us and utterly demolish us. But do you know what they saw? They saw the boys from the God-worshipers' school climbing up the posts onto the roof of that old haunted house while they were singing and whistling, "Onward, Christian soldiers! Marching as to war." That's what they saw. And one by one the pieces of thatch were thrown down. One by one the bamboo rafters were thrown down. One by one the floorboards were pulled up. One by one the posts were pulled over. By noon the whole house was torn down, and nobody's head had been crushed, nobody's arms or legs had been broken. Nobody had even gotten as much as a splinter in his finger.

The spirit worshipers could not believe it. Their devils had no power over the God worshipers! They stood in awed silence a moment, then someone shouted, "Look out! They'll eat you!" The crowd fled in panic and hid themselves in their houses. It didn't take long to load the posts and floorboards onto our wagons, and by evening the old haunted house was carted to the riverbank across from our mission station.

"Well, Thara Peter," I said. "How are we going to get this lumber across the river?"

"Oh, that's easy, Dr. Rabbit," said Thara Peter with a smile. "All we need to do is to tie it together into a raft, and then pull it across the river with our motor launch. The posts are too heavy to float by themselves, but the two-by-fours and the floor boards are light, and I'm sure when it is all tied together it will float enough for us to pull it across."

"Splendid, Thara Peter!" I said. "We shall do just that." The next morning we placed two big ropes in the water and carefully piled our posts and floorboards on top of them. When it was all in order, we tightened the ropes around the pile and levered it into the deep water, and it floated! The top was only about half an inch above the water, but that was enough. We tied the front rope to the back of the launch, and started the engine. I put Thara Peter at the wheel while I took care of the engine.

"Head upstream about half a mile," I told him. "Then when you start across, the current will take us down and land us right on our mission property."

All went well. We began to move. We gathered momentum. I opened up the throttle of the engine to full power. We were doing fine. Suddenly Thara Peter glanced back for a moment and saw the wave from the back of the launch going right over our raft. "Look, Doctor!" he shouted. "The water is going right over the raft! "

I looked, then smiled. "It's all right, Thara Peter. Don't worry. The raft is not sinking."

"Yes, but look, Doctor. Look!"

I looked again. "It's all right," I said assuringly. "What's the matter?" "Look, Doctor! The house is getting *baptized.*"

I smiled. "It sure is! And this is our second baptism!" That house was converted all right. We landed on the mission property right where we wanted to. In just three weeks the house was rebuilt, and each evening instead of the screaming of evil spirits you could hear Thara Peter and his twenty-six boys singing, "What a wonderful change in my life has been wrought, since Jesus came into my heart."

But more than the boards of that house were baptized. Within another year or so we baptized a brother and sister of Fair One and a little later we baptized the mother, old Rippling Water herself.

As I saw their happy faces, I said to Mamma Rabbit, ''I'm so glad we came to Burma. I feel more and more that this is our special place."

"I do too!" she whispered happily.

Dr. Rabbit Earns a New Degree

DR. RABBIT! Oh, Dr. Rabbit!" groaned a man one day as he came up the steps, holding his hand with a huge boil on the back of it. "Look, Doctor. I need some powerful fry-smell medicine to make my hand better."

"Fry-smell medicine?" I said in surprise. "What kind of medicine is that?"

"Something to drink," he explained, "that will take all the fry smell out of my hand, so it can get better."

Now, I had heard many of my patients talk about the "fry smell"—that is, the smell of any frying food—and they always seemed to associate it with the pus in sores, boils, pimples, and abscesses. I was eager to learn more about their ideas, so I asked, "What has fry smell got to do with that boil on your hand?"

"Well, you see, Doctor, it was like this," he said. "About ten days ago I was cutting bamboos in the jungle, and a piece of bamboo slipped across the back of my hand and cut it. It didn't bleed very much because I picked up a handful of dirt and rubbed it in, and it would have been quite all right, but that night when I got home my neighbor was frying a chicken and the fry smell came into my nose, went down into my stomach, came up my left side and down my left arm, and that night my hand began to throb and throb. The next day it got bigger and bigger and redder and redder, till now, just look at all the fry smell in my hand."

Oh! I thought to myself. So that's it. They think the fry smell causes infection. I smiled and said, "Uncle, it was the germs in that handful of dirt that caused that boil, not the fry smell."

He looked at me in blank disbelief as I went on. "But, anyway, I've got something better than drinking medicine for that boil of yours." I went to my cupboard, slipped a little lance up my sleeve, and came out with a bottle of iodine and a swab in my hand. I painted the iodine all over the boil then looked up quickly and pointed outside. "Oh, look, Uncle! Look at that little bird over there on the tree."

While he looked I lanced his boil. He felt me cut and turned around. There was the pus running down into the basin, yellow and brown and green, with a very bad smell. His eyes sparkled. "There it goes! There it goes!"

I said, "What goes?"

"Ah," he said, "the fry smell!" He was quite convinced that the pus was coagulated fry smell. "Now my hand will get better, won't it?"

I said, "It surely will."

His hand did get better, and that delighted man went up and down the country telling everybody he met, "If ever you get the fry smell, go down to Dr. Rabbit at the God-worshipers' sickness house. He has the last word on fry smell. He's the Fry-Smell Specialist."

"Fry-Smell Specialist!" "Why not? I thought to myself when I heard of it. Why not have a degree after my name? —Dr. Rabbit,

F.S.S.! Why not?

There followed a regular run of fry-smell patients with boils, pimples, sores, and abscesses. I treated them all to their entire satisfaction except for one thing. Naturally, being a graduate nurse from the Sydney Sanitarium, I preached the germ theory of infection, and I urged cleanliness, hot water, soap, iodine, and clean bandages for all cuts and sores. But anon I would hear them laughing and talking behind my back, "Ha! Ha! Ha! Germs! Whoever saw a germ?"

"I never did!"

"Me neither!"

"But the fry smell? Everyone can smell the fry smell."

"Of course, their medicine is powerful."

"Yes, but their ideas are sure odd!"

"Germs! Ha! Ha! Ha!"

"Whoever heard of such a thing?"

Then Dr. Rabbit got another brilliant idea. Hadn't someone said, sometime or other, "If you can't lick 'em, join 'em?" So I tried a new approach. I renamed my iodine. I called it *fry-smell medicine* and began to preach, "Paint your cuts and sores with Dr. Rabbit's fry-smell medicine; put a clean bandage around them, and that will keep the fry smell out." It worked.

I did even better than that. I adopted the picture of a rabbit for my trademark. I duplicated labels for my medicines, so that now I had Dr. Rabbit's Bunny Brand Castor Oil, Bunny Brand Ringworm Lotion, Bunny Brand Itch Powder, and Bunny Brand Fry-Smell Medicine!

But don't get the idea that it was an overnight victory. One day a worried mother came to the dispensary and begged me to come and treat her little baby who was too sick to be carried down to the dispensary. As soon as I finished the other morning patients I went up to her village in the motor launch. The baby *was* sick. I gave it one treatment, but it needed constant care for several days. I said to the worried mother, "You'd better bring the baby down to the dispensary where Mamma Rabbit will be able to care for it for two or three days. Then I am quite sure it will get better. You can come back with me in the launch."

"I don't mind if I do," she replied, and she quickly got together a small basket of rice and some clothes and followed me down to the launch with her baby. Now, you know, there is always an oily smell around all motor engines, especially when they backfire. Well, this day as I started the engine of the launch, it backfired and filled the launch with exhaust smell. The poor mother was terrified. She grabbed the baby in one arm and the rice and clothes in the other, and leaping out of the launch, away she ran, screaming at the top of her voice.

"Fry smell! Fry smell! Look out for the fry smell!" and all attempts to contact her again failed.

Another time I was called to a village about six miles away to see a sick man. I decided to go by bullock wagon and take my projector with me in the hopes of showing some pictures on the life of Christ in the evening. All went well. I visited a number of sick people. They were all excited about seeing the pictures, and when I was ready, and began to play my trumpet, they gathered together. Soon I was showing the wonderful pictures and the crowd was oh-ing and ah-ing.

Well, in those days we used carbide gas for our light. Your grandpas can tell you all about carbide gas. Small lumps of carbide are placed in a can, then water is dropped onto the carbide drop by drop. At once bubbles begin to form on the lumps of carbide and the gas is given off. It passes up through a rubber tube to the burner, where it burns with a very bright white light. But the gas has a very, very bad smell. If, as sometimes happens, there is a drop or two too much water, the gas generates too fast for the burner to burn it. Then the gas just bubbles up through the water, "doodleoodle-oodle," and you can smell the escaping gas everywhere—that very bad-smelling gas.

Well, I was maybe halfway through my pictures when I heard my generator go "doodle-oodle-oodle." It gave me no time to think. The people nearest the generator smelled the gas, and instead of asking what it was, they sprang to their feet, wrapped their shirts and blankets around their heads, and yelled, "Fry smell! Fry smell! Look out for the fry smell!" Everyone in the crowd stampeded for the jungle, and nothing I could do or say could persuade them to come back and see the rest of the pictures.

In spite of the quite frequent fry-smell disappointments, however, our reputation spread farther and farther into the jungle villages. More and more we were being called to a village where some delighted patient had told all he knew about the God worshipers and their powerful medicine. This was exactly what we had hoped for and prayed for. We discovered that we were welcome to stay in the home of every satisfied patient we had ever had, and we could hold meetings there with no opposition. What we needed now, was more workers on the staff. I needed a Karen evangelist to help do the visiting. I needed two more teachers for our growing school. I needed an associate missionary who was also a nurse, so one of us could be in the field and one could look after the home-base dispensary.

In a wonderful way God supplied the needed teachers and the evangelist almost at once. The evangelist's name was Tha Myaing, and you can read the story of his remarkable life in one of the recent MV Book Club books, *Jungle Storyteller*.

I also began to dream of someday establishing out-schools, with teachers in charge who would be trained to care for the minor ailments of the village folks. To this end, I asked one of my teachers and one of my big school girls to act as nurse's aides for two hours before school each day, a week at a time. In this way several teachers and students learned how to diagnose the common fevers and treat the various sore eyes and skin diseases common to the village folks.

As soon as Tha Myaing, the new evangelist, was settled, we went through our record sheets and made a list of the patients in the villages to the west of us. We packed the canvas bags to be carried on our backs, putting in a change of clothes, a small mosquito net, and a generous supply of simple medicines. Then we took to the road for a two-week trip.

What a thrill that trip was! In each village we visited our previous patients, to their inexpressible joy. "Dr. Rabbit has come! Dr. Rabbit has come!" they shouted. Little boys went scampering off to call their aunties and uncles and grandpas and grandmas. We were entertained with the best food the village had. We were given the best bamboo veranda to sleep on. We had a splendid meeting every evening. And as I sat with Tha Myaing and the old men around the campfire after each evening meeting, I said again and again to myself, "This is it! This is it!"

However, the trip was not without its heartaches.

"Doctor, Doctor!" cried a man as we came into a village twelve miles out. "Have you got any burn medicine?" "I surely have," I replied. "When did your little girl burn herself?"

"About seven years ago," was his surprising reply.

"Seven years ago? I don't know what I can do for a burn seven years old," I groaned. "Well, please come and have a look anyway," he urged.

So I went up the bamboo ladder into his house. I sat down on the veranda. I heard him call his daughter. In answer I heard something that sounded like a kangaroo hopping. The next minute a twelve-year-old girl was standing before me on one leg, while her father explained, "You see, Doctor, when she was a little girl five years old her dress caught fire one evening. It burned all of one leg and one side of her body and one arm. Then, because I had no medicine, and because you missionaries had not come yet, and because the government hospital was too far away, and because the burned place hurt to be exposed to the air, my little one just huddled in the corner, in the darkness, and cried. In six months her leg and her body and her arm had grown together." The father looked hopefully into my face as he pleaded, "Now, Doctor, have you some burn medicine to put on that terrible scar so that she can run and walk and play like other children again?"

''I'm sorry, Uncle," I said. "I can do nothing. But I'll give you a letter to the surgeon at the Moulmein Hospital. I know he will be able to do something."

"No! No! We are afraid of the hospital in Moulmein. It's too far away. If *you* cannot do it, then she must stay as she is."

I saw the hope fade out of the face of the twelve-year old. It brought a lump to my throat and tears to my eyes. Tha Myaing hastened to tell them of a loving living God who will make cripples walk someday—if they believed. Then we went on with heavy, aching hearts.

At last the trip was over. Tha Myaing and I were on our way home. About seven miles from our mission we came to the camp of our European district commissioner. I knew him well and greeted him warmly and sat in a chair beside him. He had quite a camp. It took two elephants to carry the tent, the folding furniture, and all the supplies. He had a cook, a valet, and an armed bodyguard of twelve policemen. "Where's the rest of your group?" he asked kindly.

"There are no others. Tha Myaing and I are alone," I replied.

"Alone? Where are your guns?"

"We have no guns."

"Hare, you must be crazy!" he said. "This jungle is dangerous. There are tigers, and sometimes bad men."

"Commissioner," I said, "we have been visiting our patients. Everyone is a friend. And every one of their nieces and nephews, their uncles and aunties, and their grandpas and grandmas is a friend. They look after us like kings in their villages and would gladly accompany us from one village to another if we needed them."

The commissioner nodded his head in understanding. "You're right, Hare. You see, with me it's different. In every case I judge I make one friend and one enemy, maybe many enemies. And so—"

"I understand," I said. "And I'm so glad I am a missionary." We chatted for a while, then Tha Myaing and I went on, unafraid.

We had hardly gotten home and had scarcely bathed and eaten when a lad came running from the dispensary. "Nurse Fair One says to come quick," he said. "They brought in a man who has been mauled by a tiger. He and his friend are log catchers. They catch logs floating down the river and tie them into rafts for the sawmills in Moulmein. Well, last night just as it was getting dark, they thought they saw a log and went after it. But it was a tiger swimming across the river. While they were turning around the tiger attacked the man in the back of the canoe. Oh, it's terrible, Doctor! Come quickly!"

In a few minutes I was at the poor man's side. It *was* terrible. With one paw the tiger had scratched the poor man's thigh, and there was a gash nine inches long right into the bone. With the other paw the tiger had scratched the poor man's knee, tearing away the muscles and the sinews. Then with both paws the tiger had seized the poor man by the ankle and had crushed his foot. "How did you get away from him?" I asked in amazement.

"Well, when the tiger opened his mouth to bite my foot, I shoved my paddle down his throat. Then roaring and howling with pain, the tiger let go and went away."

"You're a brave man," I said. ''I'll do my best for you." And I did. I sewed up his thigh and his knee; but that poor foot—it was mangled beyond repair. I soaked it and poulticed it day after day, but after a week there were definite signs of blood poisoning.

"Looks like I've got the fry smell in it," he said woefully.

I didn't feel like arguing. I nodded my head and said, "Come, I'll take you in my launch to the government hospital. I'm sure the doctor there can amputate your foot and save your life."

Reluctantly he agreed, and the next day we were at the Moulmein Hospital.

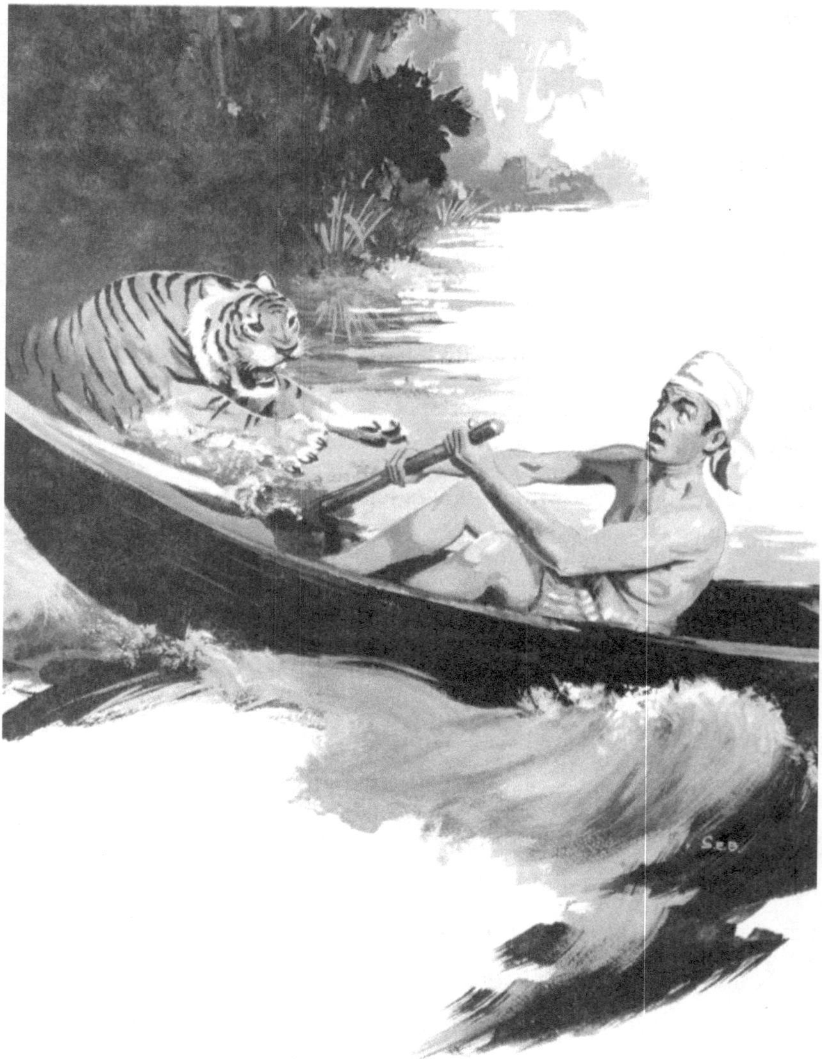

The "log" floating down the river turned out to be a tiger, and it attacked the man in the back of the canoe.

"Yes, you have brought him in time," said the doctor. "I can amputate and save his life. But first he must give his consent."

That's easy, I thought to myself, but I was wrong. The poor man listened carefully as we explained the danger he was in. But in spite of all we could say, he shook his head and said, "No, Doctor! I would rather die with two feet than go back to my village with only one foot and be a burden to my wife and my family."

In two weeks they carried him out and buried him. When we heard the sad news Mamma Rabbit looked at me with a very strange expression on her face and said, "So, Dr. Rabbit, F.S.S., there are still some cases your famous fry-smell medicine will not cure."

I nodded sadly, then added, "But for everyone that we can't help there are a *hundred* that we can. And I'm so glad we are *here*. I feel we really belong right here."

She said feelingly, "I do too."

Dr. Bear Joins Up

IT TOOK a little longer to obtain my associate missionary, but at last a fine young man, Harold Baird, arrived. He was a graduate nurse from the Sydney Sanitarium in Australia. He was also a trumpet player, and his good wife-to-be was to join us as soon as *her* nurse's course was finished. So every prospect was pleasing.

Now, the Karens have no final consonants in their speech, so when they pronounced Mr. Baird's name they had the choice of making it two syllables, "Bair-da" or of leaving off the "d" and making it "Bair." You've guessed it, they chose the latter, and because the spelling made no difference to the sound, Dr. Rabbit's new associate became Dr. Bear.

Our jungle folks were delighted, and so was I. It was now my privilege to start him off with regular language study classes. And now, as the lady doctor Mary Gibbs used to smile at *my* blunders in speech, it was my turn to smile at his innocent blunders. For example, one Sabbath morning acting as superintendent of the Sabbath school, he used the wrong tone to the right sound, and thus invited the Sabbath school to "stand and starve" instead of to "stand and sing."

It was my privilege to teach him how to lance boils and pull teeth. And now it was my turn to witness his trembling hands, to see his knees knock together, and to see the beads of cold perspiration stand out on his brow. But not for long. Dr. Bear soon passed his examinations, and I was present at his jungle graduation. It happened like this:

One morning, not many months after Dr. Bear's arrival, we were together in our dispensary during the regular morning hours. There were twenty or more patients there for treatment—Indians, Burmese, Karens; inpatients, outpatients, friends, and curious onlookers; skin-diseased, sore-eyed, fever-racked, sick, and dying; when an anxious old man pressed through the crowd and called, "Doctor! Oh, Doctor! Please come with me to see my daughter. She has burned her finger." He named a not-too-far-away village on the river, so I looked at Dr. Bear and said, "Why don't you take Fair One and the father with you in the launch, and go up and see what you can do? I'll look after the patients here."

''I'll be glad to," he said, and quickly put some picric acid solution, some ointment, and some bandages in the medicine bag-and was off.

In about three hours he was back, and I saw him and the father leading a sobbing, moaning woman toward the dispensary. "Dr. Rabbit," he said, "you didn't tell me the Karens use the same word for arm as for finger. She has burned not only her finger but also her whole arm from the elbow down. But wait, I'll start at the beginning.

"On our way up in the launch I learned that this man's daughter, Ma Thein Nyok, is an epileptic, and occasionally she has seizures. She grew up and married about three years ago. Well, last year she had a seizure and fell down with a lamp in her hand, setting fire to her baby's bed, and the little one was burned to death. After that her husband deserted her, and she had to live in her father's house.

"Well, fifteen days ago she had another seizure, and as she collapsed this time, one arm fell right into the fire.

"Well, that was bad enough. But the father was away. No one knew what to do. So the poor woman just lay there moaning on her mat with the burned arm uncared for and uncovered. Soon it began to smell. Then the flies laid eggs on it, and now her forearm is one mass of wriggling maggots! I persuaded them to come down. I think we can get rid of the maggots in a day or two, then we must try to persuade them to take her to the Paan Government Hospital to have it amputated. It's only sixty miles away."

We carefully soaked the burned arm in a diluted carbolic solution, and in two days we cleared away 200 maggots. Then we stopped counting. The relief to poor Ma Thein Nyok was tremendous, and the look of gratitude in her eyes as Dr. Bear treated her was simply pathetic.

"Now you must take her to the government hospital," said Dr. Bear to the father.

"It's too far. It would take four days in a bullock wagon. She would die before we got there."

We knew only too well he was telling the truth. I looked at Dr. Bear and he looked at me. We both looked at poor Ma Thein Nyok. With her good hand she was wiping the tears from her eyes. Poor girl!

"Have you got any ether?" asked Dr. Bear.

"Yes, we have enough," I replied slowly.

"Will you give the ether?" he asked.

I nodded and said, "Yes, if you will do the amputating."

Then he nodded.

The next day, after the morning treatments were over, we set to work. We were no trembling jungle doctors this day. Dr. Bear had been studying anatomy half the night. He knew just where the main arteries and veins were, and just where to cut. Fortunately, I had taken a short course in simple anesthesia sometime before, and I also knew what to do. Soon the instruments were all ready, and we were white-clad and confident. We had a short prayer and then came the operation.

One hour and fifteen minutes later Ma Thein Nyok groaned, half opened her eyes, and wanting to turn, groped with her good hand to ease over her burned arm. But it was not there! She groped again. She opened her eyes a little wider. For a moment she was startled with fear. Then she saw us. "Is it finished?" she asked. "Already?"

We nodded. Then she smiled and dropped gently off to sleep.

Twenty-nine days later Ma Thein Nyok went home with the bandages all off. And that was Dr. Bear's jungle graduation.

I wouldn't have you think that we were presumptuous in our efforts on behalf of our jungle patients. No, no, indeed! We sent, or took, all our appendicitis cases, gall-stone cases, bladder-stone cases, and hernias to the doctors at the government hospital sixty miles away. We were really only nurses, and we rendered only first aid. But, when we were the only ones between our patients and certain death, we certainly rendered our very best *first aid*.

Dr. Bear was much more than a jungle doctor. He was one of the most practical missionaries I have ever come across. Somewhere he had heard of people making saw pits and sawing logs into lumber by hand. When he found some big trees in the nearby forest, and big strong boys in our school, he said, "I don't see why we can't make a saw pit and saw lumber, and build a hospital and a school building and dormitories too." And he did just that.

The first building to go up was the new chapel with classrooms downstairs. The next was a duplicate dispensary building right beside the first one, to be used for inpatients.

By this time nurse Fair One had married one of our teachers, and Pink Flower, one of our own trained nurse's aides, took her place. Dr. Bear and I alternated in taking field trips with evangelist Tha Myaing, and when we were all home at the same time, Tha Myaing and I spent as much time as we could translating *Our Day in the Light of Prophecy* and writing tracts in the Karen language. Things were certainly looking up on the Karen mission station.

One morning while Tha Myaing and I were busy with our translating, one of the schoolboys rushed into my office. "Dr. Rabbit! Dr. Rabbit!" he said breathlessly. "Dr. Bear wants you at the dispensary quick! He says to tell you it's a big lady patient. She's so big he can't get her through the front double door of the dispensary. Please hurry!"

I was instantly on my way. Whatever could it be? I thought to myself as I raced along. But very soon I understood, for there in front of the dispensary, with six jungle workmen standing around her, stood a huge female elephant! "Dr. Bear! Dr. Bear!" I said. "All right! All right! And what can I do now to help you with your big lady patient?"

"Look there!" he directed, pointing to her hip. "Two months ago she was gored by a male elephant's tusk. The men thought nothing of it. But it got the fry smell, and the flies have laid eggs in it, and now look!"

"Tell the men to have the elephant lie down," he said. It took six men, shouting and yelling, to get the elephant to lie down. Dr. Bear got into action, saying, "We've got to make that hole big enough to get the hose in so we can wash it out with some carbolic solution."

It took a little time to cut a bigger hole in the elephant's hide—it was an inch thick. Then I worked the pump while he directed the flow of the solution to all parts of the swelling. I won't attempt to describe the amount or the smell of the material, or the number of maggots that came out. But through it all, Dr. Bear held up nobly. To finish up he packed in several yards of gauze dipped in iodine and said to the thankful owner, "Come again tomorrow."

He did come again the next morning, and marvel of marvels, it took only one command from the owner, and the huge patient lay down for her treatment.

"She's much better," said the owner. "She's not so nervous anymore." Dr. Bear gave the abscess another good hosing out, and said, "Come again tomorrow."

While we were at breakfast the next morning the elephant owner came running up the stairs into the house. "Have you seen my elephant anywhere?" he cried. "We gave her, her food last night at our camp three miles away. And this morning we can't find her anywhere."

"Surely no one would steal a sick elephant!" I said. "Did you look over at the dispensary?"

He ran off to look, and in a minute he was back with a big grin on his face. "She's there all right," he said, "lying under the tree waiting for her treatment!"

You may have read that elephants have remarkable memories and

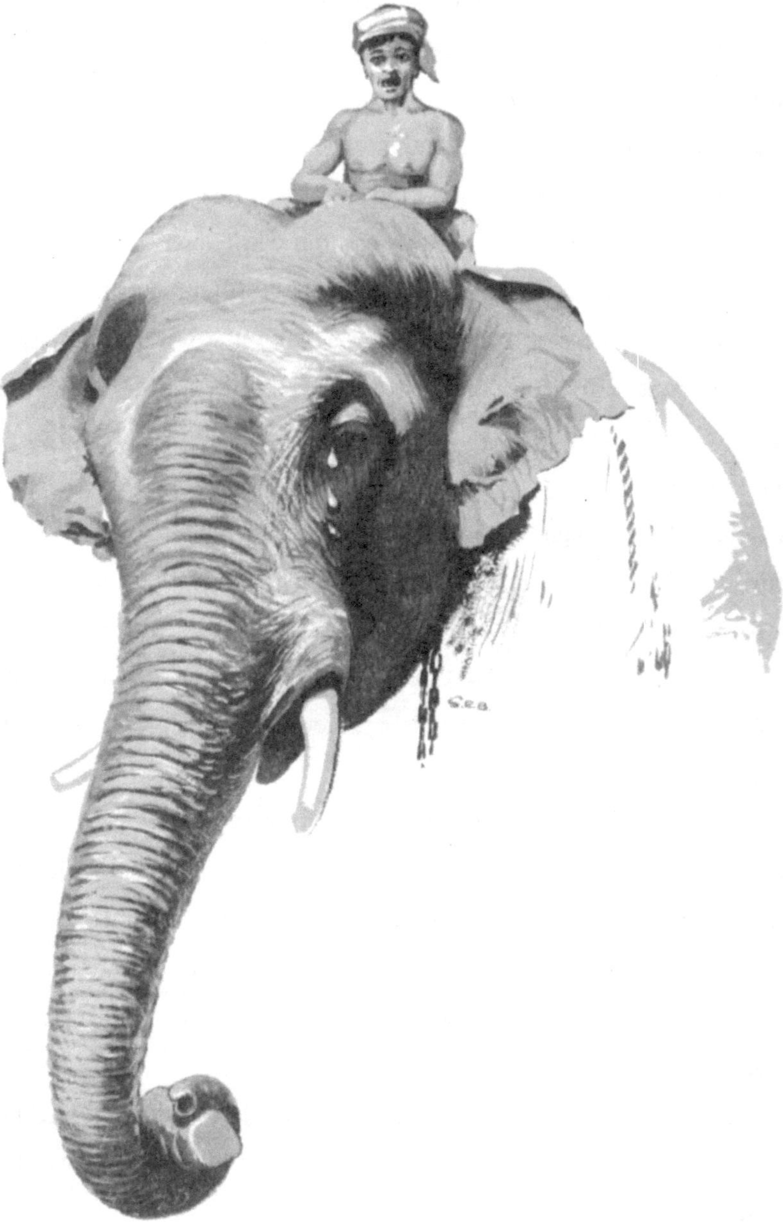

The owner mounted the elephant's head, and as the great beast took the loaf in her trunk, tears flowed down her cheeks.

are very intelligent. Take it from me, this is true. For six weeks after that Mrs. Elephant came *by herself* to the dispensary every morning and lay down *by herself* and waited for her treatment.

When the six weeks were up and the wound was all healed, the owner mounted her head and said to her, "We're going away now. Say salaam to the doctors." The big lady patient knelt down and saluted us with her trunk. I thought she deserved a going-away present, so I gave her a small loaf of bread. As she took it with her trunk and put it in her mouth (I know you won't believe this, but it's true!), tears ran out of her eyes and flowed down her cheeks! I think Dr. Bear had tears in his eyes too. I didn't look. I was too busy blowing my own nose.

Can you take another elephant story? One evening as I was working at my desk there was a sound of running and excitement outside and a man who was almost exhausted with fatigue burst through the door. Perspiration was rolling down his face and his eyes were wild with fear. "Dr. Rabbit, quick! Come quick! One of my men has been stung by an elephant!"

I knew what that meant this time, so I sprang to my feet. "Where is he?"

"In a canoe at the riverbank."

As we raced along I asked, "Where was he stung?"

The man pointed to his stomach.

"Were his bowels hurt?" I asked.

"Come and see," was all he could say.

We pushed through the reeds at the water's edge, and there on a bamboo litter, in a canoe, lay the unfortunate man. His face was pale, his breathing heavy, and his eyes closed. I lifted the blanket that covered him. The poor fellow's bowels were outside, wrapped up in his dirty loincloth. "It's too big a job for us," I whispered. "You must take him to the Paan Hospital, sixty miles farther down the river."

"We have already paddled twenty miles," said the work boss. "We are too tired to paddle another mile. He is nearly dead anyway. So if you can't do anything for him, we'll just wait here till he dies, and bury him."

Oh, what a challenge!

A small group of boys had followed us to the river's edge. I sent some of them to get the school blackboard to use as a stretcher, and one boy to go for Dr. Bear. In a very short time Dr. Bear was at my side.

The work boss was giving more details. "Today his elephant was in a nasty mood, and while the man was urging him to pull a little harder, the elephant got mad and gored him with his tusk and threw him into the air. When he hit the ground his bowels came out. We thought he was dead, but he wasn't. We waited a few more minutes, and he still lived. So we gathered up his bowels, wrapped them in his loincloth, put him in the canoe, and brought him down here to you."

"Is there any hope, Dr. Bear?" I asked. "Is there anything we can do?"

"There is no hope unless God works a miracle," said he. "But can we do *nothing* and let him die? We must at least give him first aid. Have we enough ether?"

Immediately we went into action. The poor man was carried to our operating table and we worked late into the night. We made gallons of sterile salt solution and sterilized our needles and our forceps. When all was ready, I put the man to sleep, and then I put Pink Flower in charge of the anesthetic. Dr. Bear and I washed those bowels as carefully as we could, removing every piece of dirt or leaf that we could see, and put the bowels in place again. We sewed up the gash, bandaged him up tightly, and waited for the man to come to. It didn't take long. There was a flickering of his eyes, a look of fright, a groping for the bowels, a tired smile, and the man struggled to rise, saying, "Now let me go home!"

"Not just yet," we said quickly. Then we explained that though we had done all we could, there was no human hope that he could live. He seemed to understand. We said, "We are servants of God, and we are going to pray to our living God to perform a miracle for you and let you live."

We prayed. Then we said, "Now *you* pray."

I wish you could have heard that prayer. It was so simple, so short, so earnest:

"God of the white man, make me better.

"God of the white man, make me better."

And the God of the white man heard that prayer and did make him better.

Of course, there was a lot of pus we had to keep cleaning up. For weeks we felt it was a miracle just to find the man alive each morning. But the wound finally healed! He lived! In two and a half months he walked thirty-eight miles back to his home, well and strong again. ''I'm so glad you are here, Dr. Bear," I confided.

''I'm glad I am here, too, Dr. Rabbit," he replied.

"Do you know? I feel I am needed right here."

"And do you know? I feel I am too," he said.

The Curse of the Devil Tree

"GOOD morning, Dr. Rabbit!"

I looked up from my desk and there was Dr. Bear. "Good morning, Dr. Bear," I replied. We both smiled, then I added, "And what can I do for you this fine morning?"

"We had only a few patients this morning," he replied. "So when they were finished I left Nurse Pink Flower in charge, and took a walk around our mission. You know, Dr. Rabbit, our new buildings look great!"

"They certainly do!" I agreed enthusiastically. "The chapel and classrooms, the girls' dorm, the boys' dorm, and now the new hospital. Dr. Bear, we can never thank you enough. What would we have done without you?"

"Oh, I know the buildings look good," he admitted modestly, "but I've just been looking at our rough desk tops in the classrooms and the rough table tops in the dining room."

"They were the best we could make at the time," I said.

"Yes, you had boards only six inches wide then," he replied. "But, Dr. Rabbit, if I could find a big tree that would make boards twelve inches wide, so that we could put nice new tops on our desks and dining-room tables, what would you say to that?"

"Why that would be marvelous, Dr. Bear," I said heartily, "but where are you going to find a tree big enough for that?"

"Well I've looked everywhere on this side of the river," he admitted, "and there is nothing here, but, Dr. Rabbit, across the river there is a huge tree lying on the ground, on the side of the hill where Rippling Water's son Ton Pey planted his rice last year. It is five feet through at the butt. It is thirty-three feet long up to the first fork, and it is three feet through there! It is solid all through and it would make plenty of magnificent boards twelve inches wide."

"But, Dr. Bear!" I interrupted seriously. "Don't you know? Haven't you heard? Hasn't anyone ever told you?"

"Told me what?"

"Why, that's the old devil tree of the Village of Thirty-three Pagodas! And it's supposed to be cursed!"

"Cursed?"

"Yes, cursed! Here, Dr. Bear, sit down and I'll tell you about it," I said. So he sat down and I told him the story.

"You see, years ago there was a village over there called the Village of Thirty-three Pagodas, because it had thirty-three pagodas on the ridge of hills at the back of it. Well, about 1885, when the British annexed Upper Burma, the people of that village got scared of the white man's 'thunder sticks' and 'lightning sticks' (their firearms) so they moved back into the hills of Siam. Now this tree you have been telling me about was their devil tree, where the evil spirits responsible for sickness and all kinds of bad luck lived. And offerings of bananas, tobacco, betel nut, and rice were placed in a little spirit house at the foot of that tree every day. Well, before moving away, the headman took a diamond, and making a cut in the bark somewhere, he inserted the diamond in the heart of the tree and uttered this prayer:

" 'O Spirit of the Forest,
We have lived here for many days,
But now we are going away,
And we do not want anyone else to live here.
So here is an everlasting offering for you.
Watch over this place and keep it for us
In case we might come again.
Curse anyone who will try to build a village here.
Curse anyone who tries to steal this diamond from your heart,
Yea, curse him with sudden death.'

"The story was told for miles around, and afraid of the curse no one ever dared to come near the old devil tree, or to build a house anywhere near it. Years went by and the devil tree grew bigger and taller. When we built our mission station on this side of the river the old devil tree was the most outstanding on the other side. Our schoolboys who searched all through the jungle for eatable roots and bamboo shoots said you could easily find the brick ruins of the thirty-three pagodas on the top of the ridge. So it looks as though the story is true. Well, they say that a few years before our mission station was built, in a village a few miles away, two men got their heads together and said, 'Look, many years have gone by and nothing ever happens. It is evident that the curse of the old devil tree has no more power. Come, let us saw it down and split it up and look for the diamond.' So they took their axes and their saw to the old devil tree and they sawed, and sawed, and sawed, and sawed. They must have been about halfway through when suddenly one man straightened up and cried out, 'I can't work anymore! I'm sick! Take me home! Take me home!' His workmate carried him home and in a few days he was dead!"

"Oh, ho!" said Dr. Bear. "So that's the story of the curse of the old devil tree!"

"'I'm not half finished yet," I said. "A few more years went by. We built our mission station here. Fair One, our first dispensary nurse, was baptized. Her mother, poor old Rippling Water, was driven out of her village, and then one day she came to me and said, 'Dr. Rabbit, two more of my children Naw Too and Ton Pey want to be baptized next camp meeting, and I've been thinking. If you baptize my children and baptize my house, maybe I should learn more about God and be baptized too.'

"And I said, 'Wonderful!' Then she said, 'But it's no use getting baptized unless I understand, and I can't understand unless I hear the preaching, and I can't hear the preaching unless I live close enough to come.'

" 'That's right, Rippling Water,' I agreed. 'So where do you want to live?'

" 'I would like to build my new house just across the river,' she said, 'where the Village of Thirty-three Pagodas used to be. Then I could come to Sabbath school and church every Sabbath.'

" 'Splendid, Rippling Water!' I agreed. 'Some of the big boys and I will help you build your house.'

"Then she lowered her voice to a whisper and said, 'Yes, but, Dr. Rabbit, what about the curse of the old devil tree? Does it have any power over Christians?'

" 'Indeed, no!' I replied. 'Look at us over here right beside the haunted, cursed pagoda! Nothing ever happens to us. Heathen curses have no power over Christians.'

"Her face brightened up with a big smile. 'Then I will,' she said. 'I'll build my house just across the river.' And she did. And Ton Pey lived with his mother and came across the river every day to school.

"Then one day Ton Pey stepped into my office and said, 'Dr. Rabbit, I've been thinking of clearing the side of the hill where the old devil tree is, to plant my rice this year. Now I'm not going to fool around with the old devil tree, but if I fell my trees and bamboos toward the old tree, and if, when they are dry and I burn them off, the fire burns down the old devil tree, could the curse do anything to me?'

" 'Indeed it could not, Ton Pey,' I replied.

" 'Then that's what I'll do,' said Ton Pey. And he did. And when the dried-up trees and bamboos burned away, lo and behold, the old devil tree lay in the ashes.

"The jungle folk were excited. 'Now watch him die!' they said. 'Now watch him die!' But Ton Pey didn't die. He planted his rice all around the old devil tree and reaped a bountiful harvest.

"Then two more men in a nearby village said, 'Ah, now the curse is certainly broken. Look! The Christian is well and strong, and he had a good crop of rice. Come on, let us go and cut the old tree up and look for the diamond.' So *they* took *their* axes and their saw and started to cut through the old devil tree just below the fork, and they sawed, and sawed, and sawed, and sawed. They must have been about halfway through, when one of the men straightened up and cried out, 'I can't work anymore! I'm sick! Take me home!' His workmate carried him home, and in a few days *he* was dead!"

I paused and waited for Dr. Bear to speak. "So that's the tree!" he said slowly. "I noticed the saw cut near the fork, about halfway through." "Yes, Dr. Bear," I said. "That's the tree, and that's the story. Now what do you want me to do?"

Dr. Bear was quiet for a moment. Then he said, "It truly is a lovely tree! And it would make wonderful desk tops and table tops!" Then he grinned and looking me straight in my eyes he said,

"Dr. Rabbit, I'm not scared! Are you? Look here, you know the government men better than I do. You get me a saw-pit license for that side of the river, and the boys and I will saw the thing up into boards."

"And what if you find the diamond?" I suggested. "So much the better," he laughed, and went away happy.

In about three weeks the saw-pit license came, and in about three more weeks Dr. Bear happily announced, "We have two fine logs, each fifteen feet long, and we have built the saw pit just down the hill a few feet from where the logs are. We will have the first log on the skids this afternoon."

I saw the excited boys pile into the motor launch with Dr. Bear that afternoon and go across the river to Rippling Water's landing. In about an hour I heard a mighty shout of triumph, and I knew that the first log had been rolled into position on the saw-pit skids. Then suddenly I heard the motor launch engine start up. I rushed out onto the veranda just in time to see them carrying somebody into the launch. "Oh, no!" I cried. "I hope no one has been hurt." There was no shouting or laughing as there usually was when the boys came back from work. I rushed down to the launch landing. "What's the matter?" I shouted. "What's the matter?" For answer they pointed to Dr. Bear who lay on the seat, white as death,

"An accident?" I questioned.

"No, Doctor. Everything went all right. The log rolled down as nice as could be, but as soon as it came to its place on the skids, Dr. Bear cried out in pain, 'I can't work anymore, boys. I'm sick! Take me home!' So we have brought him home. Dr. Rabbit, you don't think that the—"

"No! No! Of course not," I replied hastily. "It has nothing to do with the curse." But by the time we carried Dr. Bear to his home he was delirious, and that night all through the jungle the poor frightened people whispered, "The devils have got him. The devils have got him. Now we will see who is the strongest, the white man's God or our devils."

I sent one of the boys for Nurse Pink Flower. "Tell her to bring the fever thermometer," I said. And by the time we had him in bed, she was there. His temperature was 105 degrees.

"He had a chill last night," said Mamma Bear. "I tried to persuade him not to go to work today, but you know how enthusiastic he is about those logs."

"A chill last night, you said?" and I noted the time of it on my chart. "Any fever during the night?"

"Yes," she replied, "but he said he was all right this morning. So I thought it was just another attack of malaria. "

"I think it is malaria too," I said. "But you know a person can get it again from the mosquitoes, and sometimes it can become very complicated. There could be some very bad mosquitoes over where those logs are."

Fortunately, I had had a short course in giving intravenous injections, so calculating about an hour before the time he had the chill the previous evening, I injected the proper dose of quinine. However, he had other chills, and we had to follow this program for three days before his temperature came down to normal. But for ten days Dr. Bear was a very sick man. Then our mission president advised him to take a rest in our rest home in the Shan States of northern Burma to recuperate.

In three months Dr. Bear was back with us again, as good as new, hale and hearty as ever, and it was very gratifying to see the jungle folks wagging their heads and to hear them say, "Oh, well, of course the white man's God is stronger than our devils. Of course! Of course!"

Dr. Bear's illness led me to believe that the two men who died after sawing on the devil tree died of malaria. But I could never convince the jungle folks of that. They *knew* it was the curse that killed them.

Would you like to hear about the diamond we found while sawing the devil tree into boards? Well, while Dr. Bear was away recovering, we realized that these logs were too big for our boys to saw. We decided to hire some professional sawyers. One morning after my morning patients in the dispensary had been cared for, I heard a yell and a shout from across the river. Then I could hear the saw going double speed. It sounded so exciting that I sped across the river in the launch to see what it was all about. There were the men as excited as could be, the perspiration just rolling off them, their eyes bulging with expectancy.

"What is it? What is it?" I shouted.

"We—came—to something hard," panted the man on top of the log without slackening his speed. "It may be—the diamond!"

In a glance I could see that they had started the cut at one end of the log, and after going about one third of the distance, had stopped and started on the other end. Could it be that they had struck the diamond? I had thought that any diamond the headman might have inserted in the tree would be very small, maybe no larger than a grain of sand. But who could tell? They had only a few more inches to go. I was becoming excited too. I found myself putting the chocks in place to hold the log when it split open. I occupied myself getting the big wooden wedge ready to force the log open as soon as they stopped sawing. Then all of a sudden I heard the saw grating on something hard.

"There it is!" the men shouted as they carefully tilted the saw to cut as far above and as far below the diamond as possible.

"Finished!" shouted the man on top. And he quickly pulled the saw up through the saw-cut. I placed the wedge in position. The sawyer gave it a few blows with his sledge, and the great log rolled open, and there it was! No, not the diamond, but the hard thing they had hit while sawing. And that hard thing, as plain as could be, was a big thirty-bore bullet that somebody at some time or other had shot into that tree. For a moment we were awed, and a little disappointed. Then the humor of the situation struck us and we sat down and laughed to our heart's content. Of course, a very tiny diamond might still be there embedded in some of the limbs, or in some of our boards. But we didn't bother to hunt for it anymore. We were quite satisfied with the real treasure that we got from the old devil tree-brand-new desk tops and table tops! And you should have seen the grin on Dr. Bear's face as he said, "It was worth it, wasn't it, Dr. Rabbit?"

And I said, "It certainly was." And he added, "I feel the Lord surely wanted me to be here-right here—at this time, and for this experience."

And I said, "I do too."

The Witch Doctor's Magic

DR. RABBIT! Dr. Rabbit!" the headman of a nearby village whispered hoarsely. "Please feel my stomach."

Dr. Bear and Tha Myaing were out on tour, and I was caring for the home base. One glance at the headman showed me that he had lived a very dissipated life. His body was swollen and his bleary eyes bugged out, stamping his face with stark fear.

"What's the matter with your stomach?" I asked kindly as I helped him onto the examining table.

"Lumps!" he whispered. "See if I've got lumps!"

I felt around gently and carefully, expecting maybe to find tumors or signs of cancer. But I found nothing that I could recognize. I said, "It feels all right to me, my friend. But look, you're drinking too much. You would improve in health very much if you would leave off all alcoholic drinks."

"That's what they all say." He almost wept.

"And," I went on, "if you are still anxious about lumps in your stomach, go down to the Moulmein Hospital and have them—"

"I've been there, Dr. Rabbit," he whispered. "They said they could find nothing. They too told me to stop drinking. But I know there is something." He paused and looked around to make sure we were

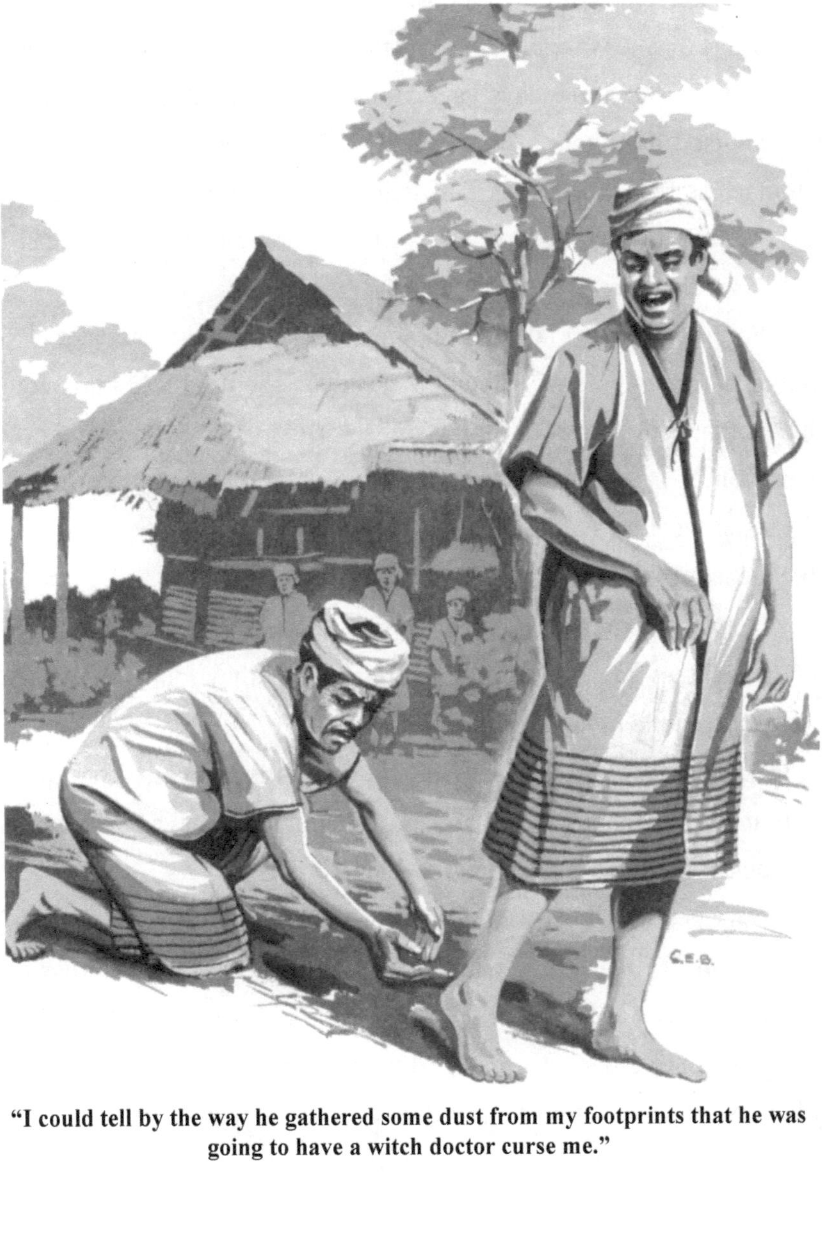

"I could tell by the way he gathered some dust from my footprints that he was going to have a witch doctor curse me."

alone. Then he whispered, "I've been bewitched! I am bewitched, I tell you! Last year I quarreled with a man in a village not far away, and I could tell by the way he gathered some dust from one of my footprints that he was going to have a witch doctor curse me. I laughed at him then, but a few days later someone whispered to me, 'You've been cursed. Two lumps of meat and a lump of rice will grow in your stomach and you will die. No medicine will save you.' I couldn't help being afraid then. I couldn't sleep unless I drank heavily. How can I stop drinking? I'm afraid! I'm afraid!"

For half an hour I talked with him about lumps that could come to anyone, even people who lived the way they should. I told him about lumps that could be taken out by surgery. But as I talked the cold perspiration of frozen fear stood out all over him. He sat up, got to his feet, and went away, the picture of forlorn misery, whispering, "I'm bewitched, I tell you. I'm bewitched!"

In just two months he died. Curiosity led the people to cut him open, and they say that in his abdominal cavity they found *two lumps of meat* and *one lump of rice!*

When I heard the news I said to Nurse Pink Flower, "I am quite convinced that that man died of fear. The lumps may have been caused by cancer, but the lumps did not kill him."

"Our people live in continual fear," Pink Flower agreed. "Fear of the evil spirits, fear of the witch doctors. Nearly every village has its witch doctor, an old, old grandpa or an old, old grandma. All they need is a little bit of a person's food and water, or part of his clothing, and, of course, a generous present, and they can utter a curse and send it on the evil wind, and that person will suffer."

"And is there no escape?"

"If the cursed one recognizes it in time, he can go to a more powerful witch doctor with a bigger present, and sometimes a curse can be reversed. But look! Here comes Fair One. She can tell you."

I looked up and sure enough there was Nurse Fair One. "So you have had experience with evil spirits and witch doctors!" I said with half a smile.

"Yes, I have, Doctor," she said. "But not since I have been baptized. Doesn't the Bible teach that Jesus and the good angels are much more powerful than Satan and his angels?"

"So you think the witch doctors are servants of Satan?"

"I do."

"And the evil spirits are the fallen angels?"

"I do. We can't see them, but they are very real. I remember one night my mother woke up choking and struggling. I said, 'What's the matter, Mother?' and she said, 'The evil spirits are after me! They demanded a pig sacrifice and I said that was too much trouble. Then I felt their icy fingers going around my throat. They squeezed tighter and tighter till I would have died if I had not agreed.' And, Doctor," Nurse Fair One continued, "the next morning mother was still angry with the evil spirits. As she put the usual small plate of rice on the spirit altar she muttered, 'There you are, you good-for-nothing spirits, always making me go to a lot of trouble.' And can you believe it? The plate of rice was thrown right back in her face!"

"Oh, ho! So that's the way they treat you!" I said.

"Yes," said Fair One. "It's no wonder the people are afraid of them. Did you hear about Uncle Big One's wife?"

"No."

"Well, you know that Uncle Big One's two boys, Little Egg and Youngest Child, have been in school for several years."

"Sure, I know. And Little Egg and his father were baptized at the last camp meeting."

"Well," said Nurse Fair One, "the mother, Uncle Big One's wife, was at the camp meeting too, and Little Egg and his father begged her to become a Christian also, but she said, 'I'm afraid the evil spirits will be angry with me.' Uncle Big One said, 'After we are baptized the evil spirits have no more power over us. Look at the Christians here; they have no fear of the witch doctor's curses, the evil wind, or even the fry smell.' But still Uncle Big One's wife said, 'I'm afraid.' Well, when they went home Uncle Big One kept on trying to persuade his wife to become a Christian, and one day she said, 'Maybe I will.' The next day she said, 'No, I'm afraid.' The next day she said, 'Maybe I will.' Well, that day Uncle Big One was visiting in the headman's house not far away when they heard screaming and the sound of beating coming from Uncle Big One's house. They ran to the house and found Big One's wife dead, with terrible black-and-blue welts all over her head and body. She had been beaten to death by the evil spirits!"

"Do you believe that, Fair One?" I asked seriously.

"Well," she shrugged, "that's what they say."

The next time I saw Uncle Big One I asked him about it. "It's true," he said sadly.

"Say, Pink Flower," I called a few days later while I was examining a carbuncle on a man's back. "What do you make out of this?" I pointed to a hopscotch pattern tattoo on the man's back, with various numbers and letters in the little squares.

"Oh, that is some witch doctor's magic medicine," she said. "Maybe it is to make him knife-proof or bullet-proof or curse-proof or snake-proof. There are all kinds. Don't you remember the dirty strings with the dirty pennies tied to them that Me-Me had tied all over her when she first came to school?"

"I remember."

"Well, they were devil charms too, supposed to keep the evil spirits away."

"And do the charms ever work?"

"It's hard to say. They tell of one man who was tattooed for protection against knife cuts. 'See if you can cut me!' he boasted to a friend. 'Go on. Here, take this sword and see if you can cut my arm off.' After a lot of persuasion the friend at last lifted the sword and brought it down with all his might. The next second, part of the man's forearm was lying on the floor. The friend fled in terror, and the man who was tattooed bled to death."

"What did the witch doctor say?"

"He said the unfortunate man must have smelled the fry smell or touched iron or eaten something sour before the tattoo had healed up!"

"Oh!"

"Only once have I heard of a witch doctor doing anything good for anyone," said Pink Flower. "When was that?" I said. "Do you remember when they brought Clever Queen down for Mamma Rabbit to treat? Well, it was a witch doctor who encouraged the relatives to bring Clever Queen here. He divined with the chicken bones and said:

" 'I see footsteps going to the north, but they don't come back.

"'I see footsteps going to the east, but they don't come back.

" 'I see footsteps going to the west, but they don't come back.

" 'I see footsteps going to the south, and *they* come back.'

"Now," Pink Flower explained, "our dispensary is to the south of their village. So the relatives came south, and sure enough Clever Queen did get better. Her footsteps did go back, and now here she is in school and going to be baptized someday!"

I said, "Maybe the witch doctor thought the mother and the grandma would be too scared to come to the God-worshipers' dispensary. Then if Clever Queen died, he would say, 'Well, I told you to go south, but you didn't go.' "

Pink Flower said, "Maybe. Or maybe the evil one thought Clever Queen would lose her *kalar* here, or that the *dawtakas* would eat her up."

"*Kalar?*" I said. "But, Pink Flower, isn't a person's *kalar* just his shadow?"

"It's more than that, Dr. Rabbit. You know when you dream at night, and you see this and see that, and do this and do that, and go here and go there?"

"Yes."

"Well, they say it's your *kalar* that does all those strange things. If a person's *kalar* ever gets lost, and he doesn't dream anymore, then all kinds of trouble can come to him. Haven't you seen the patients walking backward to the front gate, waving something in their hands? And haven't you heard them saying:

" 'Come back, *kalar,* come back. This way, *kalar*, this way. Come with me, kalar, come with me.' That's what they do to make sure their *kalar*s don't stay here in the dispensary."

"Oh!"

"And that's why they like Dr. Rabbit's medicine. They say it has strong *magic*; that's why it can overcome the fry smell and all the evil winds."

Magic! How long would it be before they could understand that all our success was because of the blessing of a kind and loving God?

One morning about this time a man came hurrying up the steps and into the dispensary. "Dr. Rabbit," he whispered, "my wife is the victim of some kind of evil wind. She can't walk and she has no appetite. We have no enemies. I don't think she has been bewitched. She hasn't eaten fried foods for months. It can't be the fry smell. Maybe she has lost her *kalar*."

"Where is she?" I asked. "They are bringing her," he replied quickly as he pointed down the path.

I looked, and sure enough there were two men carrying the poor woman in a blanket suspended from a bamboo pole. I pointed to a place where they could put her down. I took her pulse, noted her breathing, lifted one leg and noticed that the foot dropped limply, lifted a forearm and saw that the hand dropped limply also. It was a typical case of beriberi (malnutrition).

"Did your rice get wet while you were threshing it last season?" I asked.

"Yes, the man replied. "It rained hard for three days, and of course our rice was sopping wet. But after the rain we spread it out to dry. It dried all right. It has a little musty smell, but we can eat it all right."

"Tell me, would that rice grow if you planted it?"

"No, oh, no!"

"You see," I said. "Your rice is dead rice, Uncle! Your wife must have living rice to eat in order to get better." This was the only way I could explain vitamin deficiency to him. "Don't get discouraged. It may take a long time."

At once Mamma Rabbit got into action. Rice bran water to drink, and fresh vegetable and fruit juices with massage every day soon had the woman feeling much better. In ten days her fever was gone and she was eating well. We assured her that in a few months her paralysis would disappear.

Then one morning I saw an old man squatting beside her. He was muttering some kind of incantation and drawing figures on a bamboo tray with a piece of charcoal. I recognized at once that he was a witch doctor. While I was wondering what I should do I heard him say, "Yes, it's quite plain. The spirits have caught her *kalar*. It is in a village thirty-eight miles away where she was visiting her father last summer. She cannot get better until she has taken part in a spirit sacrifice in her father's village." Having given his verdict, the old witch doctor got up and began to leave with the woman.

"Don't go!" I pleaded. "She is making good progress."

"But the Ancient One has spoken, Doctor, and we must go."

"But she is in no condition to be carried so far," I urged.

"Doctor, I promise you, when we have fulfilled the demands of the spirits, I will bring her back. I promise you I will."

He never brought her back. The poor woman died on the way to their appointment with the evil spirits.

"My baby! My baby!" cried a worried mother one day. "Look at it, please, Mamma Rabbit. Look, it can't hold its head up! It can't suck very strong! When it sleeps its eyes are only half shut! There is no strength in its little arms or legs! Do you think it has lost its *kalar*? Has some evil wind blown upon it? Or has some evil person bewitched it?"

I was so glad I had Mamma Rabbit to look after the babies. I saw her take one good look and then shake her head as she said, "Another baby beriberi case." Mamma Rabbit had had fairly good success with beriberi babies. This was in the days before we had vitamins of every kind all ready prepared for old and young. She went bravely to work with what we had. In addition to giving the baby bran water, fruit juices, and cod-liver oil with malt extract, she worked on improving the mother's health and the mother's milk. Sometimes she even succeeded in borrowing some healthier mother to feed the baby for a month or two. But frequently she would come to me and say, "Dr. Rabbit, we need a supply of fresh yeast for vitamin B. We need fresh yeast! That's what we need." We had experimented with yeast powder and yeast tablets from the city, but in our hot moist climate they soon lost their power and wouldn't work anymore.

''I'm going to ask the local bakers what they use," she said, somewhat frustrated one day. She went to Kamamaung village with Pink Flower and came back with a big grin on her face and something bubbly in a small jar.

"Well, I think I've got it," she said. "It is yeast, all right, made from the juice of a bud cut off a toddy palm." And it did work! It was like magic. Mamma Rabbit then tried juice from the bud of a coconut palm, and it worked! All through the land the news spread. "Magic!

Magic! Mamma Rabbit has magic medicine for the evil wind!"

Maybe that's why some dear souls began to think that Dr. Rabbit had other magic medicines also. For one morning among the usual crowd of patients there came a little Indian woman, the wife of the Indian milkman in Kawkeyet, just one mile to the north of us. She waited patiently till all the others had been treated, then whispered, "Doctor, I want some medicine for my husband."

"Does he have fever?"

"Oh, no! No!"

"Does he have a boil or an abscess?"

"Oh, no! No! It's not that kind of sickness."

"Then what can it be?"

"My husband doesn't love me anymore. I want you to give me some medicine that I can sprinkle on his food, so that when he eats it he will love me again."

Poor little woman! My heart ached to help her. Would it be possible to explain the real magic that accompanies forgiveness, and the words ''I'm sorry"? There must be something to put on his food. I looked into her eyes for a long minute and prayed in my heart, "Help me, Father." Then the answer came. *You* may not think that I did, right, but I went to my medicine cabinet and selected the bottle of potassium permanganate. I took an eight-ounce bottle and filled it with water. Then putting the bottle on the table in front of the little woman I took just two of the crystals and dropped them into the bottle of water. Immediately the water turned red as wine. Her eyes popped wide open. "Now," I said, "listen carefully. You go home and cook your husband a meal of his most favorite food. Then before you put his greens on the table, soak them a little while in this red magic medicine. Then shake off all the medicine so he can't see it, and put it on the table." I lowered my voice to a whisper and added, "Mamma Rabbit does that to my greens every day!" (This was perfectly true, for we dared not eat greens in the tropics unless they had been soaked a little while in permanganate to kill the germs.) Then I went on. "But that's not all. You must say the magic words too."

"The magic words?" Her eyes opened wide.

"Yes! You see, maybe you did something that you can't remember that made your husband angry. So after he has eaten his favorite food and the greens dipped in this magic medicine, you must say these two magic words: 'I'm sorry.' They are very important. Then—then I am sure your husband will love you again."

It worked!

The next day husband and wife came down to the dispensary together, all smiles. They brought me a present of a rooster, which is the usual fee for a witch doctor's magic potion.

Mamma Rabbit's Baby Patients

IT MUST have been nearly midnight one Saturday night. We were sound asleep. Was I dreaming? Or did I really hear a faint *tap tap tap tap* on our back door? I turned over and listened. Then it came again, a little louder, *tap tap tap tap*. I opened my eyes. It couldn't be a dream. I was awake now. The tapping came again, followed by a soft, pleading man's voice, "Mamma! Mamma! Oh, Mamma Rabbit!"

"Who's there!" I called out. "Me! Hla Baw, one of your teachers," came the answer.

"Is something the matter?" I inquired. By this time Mamma Rabbit was wide awake and she heard the answer clear and plain.

"Ngwe Sein needs Mamma I think—right now!" "Of course Ngwe Sein needs me," said Mamma, jumping out of bed and getting dressed quickly. "She's been expecting her baby any time for several days now."

Then calling out a little louder she said, "Hla Baw, go back quickly. Light a fire, and make some hot water. I'll be over in just a minute." And as Hla Baw's footsteps raced down the back stairway, Mamma said to me, "I may be there for the rest of the night. This is her first baby, and you can never tell. If I am not back by morning, Dr. Rabbit, could you dress Eileen and Lenny and get their breakfast?"

I assured her that I most certainly could, and she was gone.

Ngwe Sein's face broke into a glad smile as she said, "I'm sorry to call you at this hour of the night, dear Mamma Rabbit, but I know everything will be all right now that you are here. I'm not afraid anymore now."

Mamma Rabbit examined the expectant mother. She waited an hour, examined her again, then said, "Hla Baw, go and call Nurse Pink Flower. The baby will soon be here."

Nurse Pink Flower came, and in another hour a beautiful little baby boy was placed in Ngwe Sein's happy arms.

"Hla Baw, you have a lovely little son," said Mamma Rabbit.

"Yes, Mamma," said Hla Baw.

"Have you decided on a name for him yet?"

"Yes, Mamma."

"What are you going to name him?"

"Well, this morning our Sabbath school lesson was about Moses, so we will call our son 'Moses'!"

"Splendid!" replied Mamma Rabbit. She waited around another hour or so to make sure all was well, then came home about four o'clock and crawled back into bed.

"It's a lovely baby boy," she whispered, "and they are going to call him 'Moses' after Moses in the Sabbath school lesson today."

And I grunted my approval, "Good! Good!"

There came another night just like this one about two years later, and as Mamma Rabbit placed another lovely baby boy in Ngwe Sein's arms, she smiled and said jokingly, "Here's little Moses' brother—Aaron." Then turning to the father she said, "What name have you chosen for this little baby boy, Hla Baw?"

Hla Baw replied, "*You* have named him already, Mamma."

"What have I named him?" asked Mamma Rabbit.

"You named him 'Aaron' just now," he said, "and Aaron it shall be." And Aaron it was.

And more or less this is the way it was with Barnabas and Stephen, Joshua and Caleb, Solomon and James, Esther and Betty, and Phillip and Paul. There was a call in the night. Mamma Rabbit was gone from her own children and her own home for hours, to bring into the world a new generation of Seventh-day Adventists. Is it any wonder that everybody loved Mamma Rabbit?

But Mamma Rabbit's calls were not limited to birthdays. The little ones suffered also with stomachache, malaria, coughs, and worms. We never have discovered why these little aches and pains always seemed so much worse at night. But it didn't take the young mothers long to discover that Mamma Rabbit's arms had a magic about them, and her words were so full of wisdom and comfort that all they needed was her presence and all was well again.

I remember well the night we heard a baby crying. It cried and cried and cried. "Can you hear that baby crying?" whispered Mamma in my ear.

"Yes," I whispered back.

"Sounds like a hungry cry to me," said Mamma.

"How can you tell?" I asked.

"I just know," said Mamma. "I'm going over to see what the matter is." And she got up and dressed and went. She was back in about an hour. "I told you it was hungry," she said. "The poor mother's breast has an abscess and hurt too much for the baby to nurse. But it didn't take long to make up a bottle of milk, and you see the baby isn't crying anymore."

"That's right. The baby isn't crying anymore," I agreed. "But tomorrow, Dr. Rabbit, I think you ought to lance that abscess. I'm sure it is ready."

I said, "All right, I can do that much for you and your babies." And I did. And in a few days both mother and baby were happy again.

Mamma Rabbit's most horrible cases were the babies who had worms. Not little pin worms, but worms as big as earthworms, six to eight inches long. How would you feel if you saw a little two-year-old baby gagging on a worm six inches long in its mouth! How would you feel if you saw a big worm wriggling out of a little child's nose! I don't know what medicines the doctors use now to get rid of worms, but we lived in the castor oil age, and we found that a big dose of castor oil, followed by a dose of Santonin powder, and later by another dose of castor oil surely produced results. And those results were nothing short of miraculous. Mamma Rabbit would take one look at a listless little four-year-old, with half-closed eyes and a distended stomach. She would say one word, "Worms," then get to work. After passing fifty to two hundred horrible worms, the child was put on regular doses of cod-liver oil and in three or four weeks you would be astonished at the improvement.

"Mamma! Mamma!" the happy mothers would cry as they came back to show her their little ones. "Look at them now! Aren't they beautiful! Oh, Mamma Rabbit, they surely would have died if you hadn't cared for them."

And Mamma Rabbit's heart would beat so fast with joy that glad tears would well up in her eyes.

There were some other horrible cases that did not end so well. There was the little three-year-old girl whose dress caught fire while she was warming herself one day. And before they could put the fire out, it had burned the skin right off the front of her legs, her stomach, her chest, and even her chin. They brought her to us right away and we did all we possibly could with wet dressings of picric acid solution, and soothing ointments. For three months she hovered between life and death. For three months we hovered between hope and despair. Then she died. Her parents wept openly, unashamed of their honest tears. And so did we, especially Mamma Rabbit. Yes, indeed, many cases made her dear heart ache.

I remember well the day that little Joshua was bitten by a scorpion. Joshua was the first-born of Fair One and Thara John. He was a fine little fellow. When he was about a year old a big black scorpion with a body one and a half inches wide, and a tail two inches long, came up between the cracks of the bamboo floor where little Joshua was playing. It stung him on the left heel, and Joshua screamed with the pain of it. Fair One was nearby, and as she turned toward her little son she saw the monster scorpion. Almost instinctively she picked up a piece of wood and killed the horrible thing. She had been a nurse in our dispensary long enough to know what to do. She tied a handkerchief tightly around little Joshua's ankle and sent one of the school children that happened to be near, to call me. "Go to the dispensary and tell Dr. Rabbit to come quick," she said. "Tell him a big black scorpion has bitten little Joshua on the heel."

As the little messenger relayed the message to me, I snatched up a lance, some iodine, and a bottle of permanganate crystals, and ran over to Fair One's house for all I was worth. "I've never treated a scorpion bite before, Fair One," I admitted, "but I'll do the same for it as we do for a snake bite." And I did. I painted it with iodine. Then I cut it two or three times right over the place where the sting was, to make it bleed. Then I sucked it hard for several minutes, and finally rubbed permanganate crystals into the cuts. Poor little Joshua screamed and screamed, till he finally fell asleep from exhaustion. He woke up again in an hour or two, then Mamma Rabbit took over. She soaked the little foot in hot salt solution. She put a poultice on it hoping that that would help to draw out some more of the poison. It might have helped a little. In fact it might have been what saved his life. But in spite of all we could do a big red swelling persisted all around little Joshua's foot. Mamma Rabbit kept up the soaking and the poulticing, but the next day the swelling had moved up to the calf of his leg. The next day it was around his knee. The poor little boy screamed continually, and only slept when he was exhausted. The next day it was in the area of his thigh, and the next day in his hip. The baby boy was getting weaker and weaker, and we began to despair of saving his little life.

That evening just as darkness was falling, Thara John knocked on our door. As I opened the door to greet him, I noticed his face was haggard and pale. His eyes were wide with fear. "Come in, John," I said. "No! No! Dr. Rabbit," he said nervously, "you come out and listen!"

I stepped out and listened. There was the usual background noise of crickets and other noisy jungle bugs, but more than that I could hear only the night cry of a small bird, *ca-ah, ca-ah, ca-ah*, in falling cadence something like the sound from an "E" to a "C' on the piano. It sounded plaintive and uncanny.

"What is that?" I asked.

"It is the call of a little night owl," said John.

"Oh!" I said. "Is that what you wanted me to hear?"

"Yes, Doctor. It is a small owl, but the jungle people call it a *Teh-preh*." "And what kind of a thing is that?" "A *Teh-preh* is a spirit catcher," said John, his voice trembling noticeably, "They say that little owl can smell death coming. And when it smells death it sits in a tree nearby and cries *ca-ah, ca-ah, ca-ah*, waiting for the spirit to depart."

"But, John, you don't believe—"

"No! no! We don't believe it is waiting for little Joshua's spirit. But the sound is so mournful, so fearful. It makes us afraid. I don't like to make this request, but Fair One made me come and ask if Mamma Rabbit would please come and sleep with us tonight?"

As you can imagine, Mamma Rabbit had heard every word. It took her only a minute to give me and the children instructions for going to bed and getting up in the morning. Then she walked off with John into the dark night. And up in the tree near John's house we could hear the little owl calling *ca-ah, ca-ah, ca-ah*. It gave me goose pimples to hear it. All night long that bird called *ca-ah, ca-ah, ca-ah*, and only the noise of the new day blotted out the doleful sound.

"The red swelling is getting up near little Joshua's heart now," reported Mamma Rabbit at breakfast time. "It doesn't look good to me. I couldn't do much, but the fact that I was there with them sharing their worries and their fears seemed to comfort them. I must sleep there again tonight."

That morning we prayed for little Joshua at worship. That evening we prayed for him again.

That night Mamma Rabbit went to sleep in little Joshua's house again. And that night the little owl—the *Teh-preh*, the spirit catcher—cried again, *ca-ah, ca-ah, ca-ah.*

Something woke me just after midnight. What was it? No one had knocked on the door. No one had called my name. I sat up in bed, wide awake, and listened. All was quiet. I listened for the haunting *ca-ah, ca-ah, ca-ah* of the little owl, but it had stopped! I knew now what had wakened me up. In spite of what I believed and what I didn't believe, I found myself wondering whether little Joshua had passed away. Had death claimed its little victim? Or maybe little Joshua had passed the crisis and was beginning to get better? There was only one thing I could be sure of. That doleful little owl had flown away. All was quiet again!

I was just beginning to wake up in the early morning when Mamma Rabbit burst into the room. "He's better! He's better!" she cried. "He passed the crisis just after midnight last night. The red swelling is moving downward, away from his heart. And he is hungry and sleeping normally again."

"I knew it!" I said. "I knew it!"

"How could you know it? Did anyone come and tell you?" demanded Mamma Rabbit.

"No. Nobody came, but the little owl stopped crying *ca-ah, ca-ah, ca-ah*, and flew away. So I just guessed that our old enemy death had gone away too," I said.

"Oh, you old jungle man!" said Mamma Rabbit with a big grin.

"Do you believe that stuff too?"

"Well, you know some things are very queer," I suggested.

But now listen! You may find it hard to believe what I have to tell you now. But by the tenth day, that big red swelling had reached the heel of little Joshua's *right* foot. There it broke out in a patch of watery blisters, and then disappeared! It's true!

And so is this true—Mamma Rabbit was often tired out after an all-night adventure, but she would always smile and say, ''I'm so happy here! So happy!"

Triumphs and Defeats

"DR. RABBIT! Dr. Rabbit!" I looked out of the dispensary window and saw the head fisherman from Kawkeyet village with seventeen of his men approaching the gate.

"Good morning to you all. How many of you are sick today?" I called, half in fun.

"It's just me, Doctor. Just me," called the head fisherman. "I've got a tooth that I want pulled out."

As I took in the situation I caught the picture of a man who expected to have a big operation and had brought his seventeen men along to assist. So I straightened up and said to myself, "All right, my good man, a big operation you shall have."

I stood in the doorway and welcomed him as one chief would welcome another, then seated him on my very best seat. I stationed his seventeen men all around the room. To one I gave a towel, to another the absorbent cotton, to another a bundle of bamboo swab sticks. Another held a glass of water, another the permanganate, another the oil of cloves, and still another held my tray containing my lance and forceps. I stationed two at his head to hold his shoulders and stroke his arms. I stationed two more to hold and stroke his legs. Then I took up my position right in front of him. I called for the oil of cloves and a swab. The men holding these things stepped forward as if they had been trained all their lives to do it.

"Now open your mouth," I said.

The chief opened his mouth and pointed to the tooth. It was very loose. I could have pulled it with my fingers, but that would never do. I painted all around the tooth with oil of cloves.

"That's hot, isn't it?" I said.

"Ugh!" he grunted.

"You've had trouble with this tooth several months, haven't you?" I continued.

"Ugh! Ugh!" he agreed.

"And you haven't slept pleasantly for three or four nights?"

"Ugh! That's right." He nodded. And his confidence in me as a dentist was increasing with every grunt.

I called for my instrument tray. I selected the right forceps for that particular tooth, and with a professional flourish, took a firm hold on the offending member. At that identical moment, however, the good man suddenly noticed that his tooth didn't ache anymore. The oil of cloves was doing its magic work. So he decided not to get his tooth pulled out after all, but to buy a bottle of this magic medicine instead. Up went his two hands to grasp my hand and prevent the pulling till he could explain, but as he jerked my hand, the tooth came out! With another flourish I gave the tooth to the man with the towel and told him to take it home, dry it, and hang it by a string on the back of the door for a souvenir. Then I dropped two crystals of permanganate in the glass of water, and had the patient wash out his mouth.

I can't remember seeing a more pleased patient in all my life. All the way home he showed everybody that he met the place where the tooth had been, and told everyone that Dr. Rabbit was the greatest dentist in the whole wide world. The next day he sent me a present of a big fish that must have weighed fifteen pounds, and on his history sheet I wrote, "Paid in full."

It may have been a week or a month after this elating experience, that another dear old man knocked on the dispensary door one morning before breakfast and said, "Dr. Rabbit, I want to get a tooth pulled out."

"Where do you live?" I asked. He named a village ten miles away. He had walked ten miles before breakfast to get his tooth pulled out! It must have been giving him a great deal of agony. I invited him in, sat him on a stool, and began my preparation. On my silver-colored tray I placed my syringe and the Novocain. When the man saw the needle, his eyes opened wide and he said, "Oh! Oh!"

Next I placed a lance and an elevator on the tray. The man's eyes opened wider and wider, and again he said, "Oh! Oh!"

Finally I selected two forceps and put them on the tray and once more he said, "Oh! Oh!"

Then I slipped into my white doctor's coat, and said, "All right, Uncle, I'm ready now. Just open your mouth and let me get to work."

But the sight of all those instruments terrified him and he covered his mouth with both hands, shook his head and said, "Hm-hm!"

I explained that after the first prick of the needle he wouldn't feel any more pain. He shook his head harder than before, and with his mouth still held shut tight, kept saying, "Hm-hm! "Hm-hm!"

Suddenly I thought of something that might build up his confidence. I went to my cupboard and took down a small jar of dried teeth-teeth that I had pulled and put in a bottle to help convince people that I really could pull teeth. I rattled them in front of him and said, "Don't be scared, Uncle! Look, I pulled all these teeth and not one of them hurt. Now come on, open your mouth and let me pull yours."

"Hm-hm! Hm-hm!" was all I could get out of him. Nurse Pink Flower tried her hand at persuading him to open up. The other patients who were there waiting for their treatments all tried. But it was no good. The man who walked ten miles before breakfast because he *wanted* to get his tooth pulled out, walked ten miles home again with his aching tooth still in his head because he was not *willing* to open his mouth and let me pull it.

"Dr. Rabbit! Dr. Rabbit!" begged a man one morning in the rainy season. "Please bring Mamma Rabbit to see my wife. She had a hard time giving birth to her baby. The baby didn't live, and now my wife has a very high fever."

The head fisherman had brought seventeen men to assist me, and I solemnly gave each one something to do.

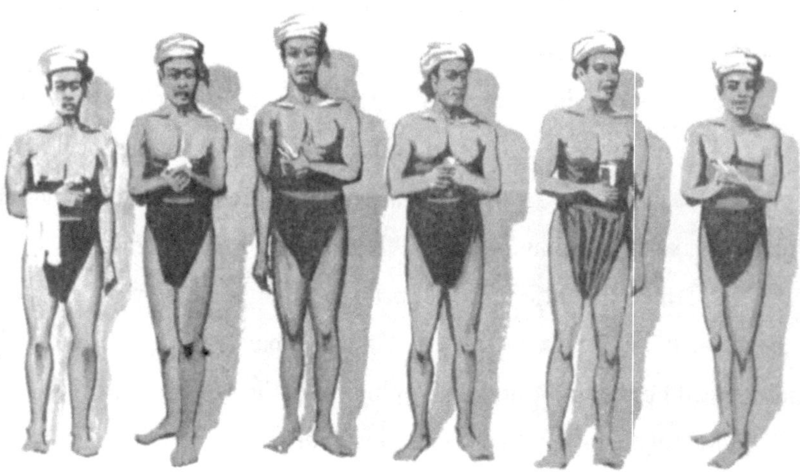

Only too well did we recognize the symptoms. Willing to do all we possibly could, we stepped into the motor launch, went two miles down the river, then walked through two more miles of the nastiest, stickiest mud to the poor man's village. As we climbed up the bamboo ladder, we noticed two or three old women sitting on the veranda with a hopeless expression on their faces. I joined them and tried to cheer them up while Mamma Rabbit and Pink Flower went inside to see the sick woman. Suddenly I realized that all was quiet inside the room. Very quiet. Too quiet!

In half an hour Mamma Rabbit and Pink Flower came out. Their faces were pale and sad. "Too late, I'm afraid," whispered Mamma Rabbit. "We have given her a treatment and have made her a little

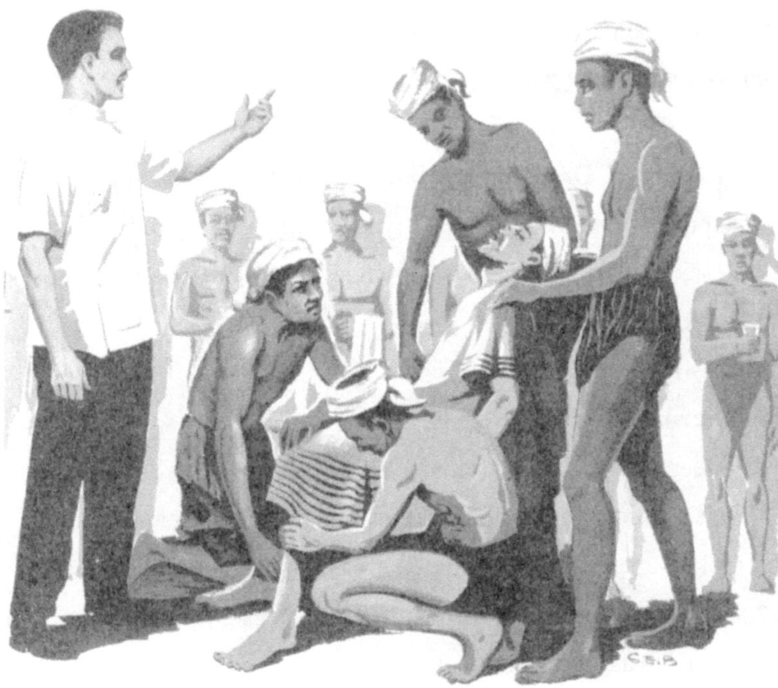

more comfortable, but the poor thing! Maybe they did their best to apply heat to her abdomen. They heated a stone, wrapped it in a blanket, and put that on her. But she didn't feel better, so they made the stone hotter, and hotter, and still hotter. Then they left off the blanket, and the poor woman has a terrible burn all over her stomach. Now it is infected."

"I wish you could have brought her to the dispensary as soon as you saw she was having trouble," I said to the husband.

"Oh, Doctor, what could we do? So many people! One saying this. One saying that. And the witch doctor saying the signs were not good. It is so far to carry a sick person through the mud." The poor man was so sad.

All the way home through the two miles of that sticky mud we were quiet. Very quiet. Too quiet. We were still quiet two days later when we learned the poor woman had passed away. And we were very sad.

"Dr. Rabbit! Dr. Rabbit!" called another man on another day. "Please put a splint on the arm of my little son, Maung Taw. He fell off the bullock wagon and the wagon wheel ran over his arm and broke both the bones."

"How long ago?" I asked.

"Fifteen days," answered the father.

"Fifteen days!" I said anxiously. "Where is he now?"

"He's coming," said the father pointing toward the gate.

I looked up and saw a twelve-year-old boy with a dirty, rag around his arm, walking painfully toward the dispensary. Suddenly I was aware that I was more than *seeing* him, I was *smelling* him, and he smelled like something dead. Gently I removed the dirty rag. There was something dead. Both of the bones between his elbow and wrist had been broken, and they poked out through the skin. The wound had become infected, and now the hand and the part of the forearm below the break were black and dead, beginning to slough away. I was horrified! But worse than that, there were definite signs of blood poisoning setting in above the break. "You must take him to the government hospital," I said definitely. "The doctor will have to amputate Maung Taw's arm."

"No! No!" pleaded the father. "We do not want to go to the government hospital. Their medicine is good, but it is not mixed with love. If the arm must be cut off, we want *you* to do it."

"If you had come fifteen days ago maybe we could have saved his arm," I argued.

"But we couldn't come till we had sacrificed to the evil spirits, and it took so long to gather the family all together. Please, Dr. Rabbit, won't you do it?"

How I wished for Dr. Bear at that moment. But I think you have already guessed it. Dr. Bear was too good a man just to be an associate missionary, and by this time he had been transferred to a new district, Shweynaung-byin, in the hill country near Toungoo. So it was just Dr. Rabbit and Pink Flower-and, of course, God too. I must not forget to mention that God was always with us.

In an hour it was all over and Maung Taw, smelling sweet as a daisy, lay smiling on his mat.

"Dr. Rabbit! Dr. Rabbit!" called a middle-aged woman on another sunshiny day, "please look at my forehead."

I looked and found she had a wen (fatty tumor) as big as a small hen's egg on her forehead. "Well," I said, "what do you want me to do about it? No medicine that we can put on that will make it disappear."

"I know," she said. "I want you to cut it out."

"That wouldn't be too hard, Auntie," I said. "But I am all out of Novocain just now. I will be going to the city for supplies at the end of the month. Come next month and I'll cut it out for you."

"Next month?"

"Yes."

"Please do it now, Doctor."

"Auntie, it would hurt a lot without Novocain."

"Hurt? Well, how long would it take you?"

"T-w-e-n-t-y long minutes," I replied with a meaningful smile.

"Twenty minutes?" she said thoughtfully. Then suddenly she lay down on the examining table saying, "All right, Dr. Rabbit, go ahead and cut. I promise you I won't move for twenty minutes."

"But it will hurt!" I objected.

"I've been ugly for twenty years," she said. "It will be worth twenty minutes' hurting to become pretty." "Do you really mean it?" I gasped. "Of course I mean it!" she insisted. "Here give me a folded handkerchief to bite on." I gave her the handkerchief. She put it between her teeth. Her hands grasped the sides of the table. She nodded her head and mumbled, ''I'm ready." For twenty minutes she didn't move while I cut that wen out and sewed up the incision. When it was over she sat up.

"Please give me a mirror," she said. We handed her a mirror. She looked happily at her reflection, then smiled and said, "It was worth it."

What wonderful people! Where else on earth could you find people like these? And just think of it! They were *our* people!

"Dr. Rabbit! Dr. Rabbit!" This time it was a little old grandma, who had waited patiently till the morning treatments were all over, then when her turn came she was speechless. She couldn't say a word.

"Do you have fever, Grandma?" I asked.

"Oh, no, no! It's not that," she managed to say.

"Maybe sore eyes?"

"Oh, no, no! It's not that."

"Ah, then maybe it's ringworm?" I named one of the most common ailments.

Oh, no, no! It's not that!"

But with this her tongue was unloosed. ''I'm starving. I tell you, I'm starving!" Then followed this heartbroken story. "My big son went to Moulmein to work in a sawmill, and he promised to send me back some money to buy rice. But he hasn't sent any money at all."

"Does he write you any letters, Grandma?" I asked sympathetically. "Oh, yes! He has written many letters, and he says he is earning good wages." "And doesn't he send *anything* in those letters?" I persisted.

"Only some crazy little bits of paper with English printing all over them!" She was angry now. "But you can't buy rice with crazy little bits of paper. You've got to have *money* to buy rice, I tell you, and I'm starving."

I was immediately suspicious about those crazy little bits of paper, so I said, "Grandma, you go right home and get all of those letters and all of those crazy little bits of paper, and bring them to me. I want to see them."

The next morning she came with the letters all wrapped up in a banana leaf. "There now," she said. "See for yourself."

I looked, and sure enough just as I suspected, every one of those crazy little bits of paper was a money order for ten rupees! "Grandma! Grandma!" I said. "Each one of these crazy little bits of paper is worth ten rupees. You just go to the post office and put your thumb print on each one, and the postmaster will give you ten rupees for each one."

For a moment grandma was too dumfounded for words, then she gasped, "I can? He will?" Hugging her letters to her heart and trembling with excitement she said, "Just to think of it! There I was starving—starving to death—with all this fortune in my hands."

As she went away rejoicing, I wondered who was the happier, she or I?

On another day there came an old man crying, "Dr. Rabbit! Dr. Rabbit! Please tie a stick on my broken thumb and put some medicine on it. I broke it when I fell out of a coconut tree ten days ago, and now it hurts so much and smells so bad."

I took off the dirty rag that covered his hand and gasped. The broken part of the thumb was black and rotting off. Blood poisoning had set in, and angry red streaks were starting up his forearm. In alarm I said, "Uncle, you must sit right down and let me cut that thumb off. It is dead. No medicine can cure that now. If you don't cut it off you will die along with it before many days."

"No, no, Doctor. Put some medicine on it," he begged.

"It's too late for medicine now," I argued. "If you had come ten days ago I could have put some medicine on it and tied it up with a stick. But it's too late now."

"No, no, Doctor! Don't cut it off today!"

I thought maybe he didn't know I could cut fingers off. So I reached up among my bottles and brought forth a finger I had cut off and had preserved in spirits. "Look, Uncle!" I said. "I cut that off, and it didn't hurt. I have the medicine to make it painless, and I have the time to do it now. Come, sit down and let me cut off that dead thumb and save your life now."

In spite of all I could say, he shook his head and said, "Not now, Doctor. Not now! There's a powerful witch doctor not far from my village. I'll go try his medicine for ten days. And then, if it's not better, I'll come and let you cut it off." Away he went. But he never came back. He died just five days later. When I heard it, I wept. I could have saved his life. I had the time. I had the medicine. But he was not willing.

But my patients were not all like that. Indeed, they were not. One day I was on tour in the village of Awbawa. Among those who crowded up into the schoolhouse for treatment there came a man groaning with pain caused by a huge abscess on his wrist. "Dr. Rabbit! Dr. Rabbit!" he cried. "Quick, get your knife and cut it. Cut it deep, and squeeze all the pus out."

"It will hurt if I do that," I said seriously.

"Never mind if it does hurt," he cried. "Come on, get your knife and cut it!"

"You're a strange man," I replied playfully. "Do you like people to hurt you?"

"No, no, of course I don't!" he said. "But I haven't been able to sleep or eat pleasantly for ten days. And I am thinking about being able to sleep again and eat pleasantly again. So come on, Doctor, get your knife."

"And you really *want* me to cut you and hurt you?"

"Doctor, why do you wait?" he cried. "Do you fear I will make too much noise, and move around too much? Then look! Call those six big men over there and make them sit all over me. Then take your knife and cut, cut deep!"

I did that very thing. I had the six big men sit all over him. On his legs, on his stomach, and on his arms. Then he gritted his teeth and said, ''I'm ready, Doctor. Now cut it."

I have already told you that I know how to lance boils. But let me add right here that I have *not* learned how to lance boils painlessly. This day as I lanced this poor man's abscess, it hurt, and he groaned with pain. "Shall I stop now?" I said half in fun.

"No, no, Doctor! Keep on till it's finished," he said. I probed and squeezed, and he groaned some more. "Shall I stop now?" I asked.

"No, no! Keep on!" he replied. I packed that abscess with a wick dipped in iodine. It was agony for him, and again he groaned. "Shall I stop now?" I asked again.

"No, no, Doctor! Keep on! Keep on!" he begged.

At last it was all over. A clean bandage covered his hand. The six big men got off him and moved away. He sat up, looked at his hand, then moved over beside me. He took my hand in his-the hand that had cut him and hurt him—and stroking it, he wept out his joy. "Oh, thank you, Dr. Rabbit! Thank you so much!"

When I got home from that tour I said to Mamma Rabbit, "We have the most wonderful people in all the world to work for, and I love them so much!"

She said, "I do too!"

I said, "And just think, we get paid for all this happiness."

She said, "Sh-h! Don't tell anyone, or we might be sent back home."

A Real Doctor Comes

"DR. RABBIT! Dr. Rabbit! My eye hurts. My eyelashes turn inward and scratch my eye till I can't stand it. I pull the eyelashes out, but they grow in again. Can you help me, please?"

I looked at the young mother's eye. It was swollen and sore. The eyelashes were indeed scratching the eyeball. But the delicate surgery that would be required to correct the condition was beyond my skill. This would not be first aid! All I could do was to say, ''I'll put your name on my list. I'm hoping for a real doctor to come to visit and to help me someday."

"Dr. Rabbit! Dr. Rabbit! I've got a lump on the outside of my stomach. Sometimes it is big; sometimes it is small. Can you please fix it for me?"

I looked at the lump. It was a hernia. I made a belt to help the man for the time being, and added his name to my list.

"Dr. Rabbit! Dr. Rabbit! I can't see out of one eye. I think it has the cold wind in it. Can you do something for me?"

I examined the eye. The poor fellow had a cataract. He said he would rather be blind than go to the city hospital. So I added his name to my list, and day-by-day, month-by-month, the list grew, and I had to be content to help the 90 per cent of the cases that were within our ability.

But I was not satisfied. Frequently I sent reports of our work and stories of our successful experiences to our division paper, the *Southern Asia Tidings*, and I often concluded my stories by saying I was longing for the day when a real doctor could come and help me with the cases that were beyond my ability. This was before we had a hospital in Rangoon. It was before we had even one real doctor in the whole of Burma.

Away over in our Gopalganj Hospital in Bengal, Dr. Schilling read those stories and his heart was moved. He said to himself, ''I'd like to go over and spend two or three weeks with Dr. Rabbit." He wrote to the division medical secretary.

"But we can't spare you," came back the reply. "Then will you let me spend my vacation with him?" he begged.

"It's up to you," was the reply. "If you'd rather spend two or three weeks with Brother Hare in the steaming jungle than rest in the beautiful hills, we won't stand in your way."

And so one happy day Dr. Charles Fredrick Schilling, L.R.C.P.S., arrived at our mission station with a big trunk of supplies and instruments. We had the brass band out to welcome him, and our choir of eighty-three voices sang to delight his heart. But Dr. Schilling had come to work, and he reported at our little dispensary the next morning with his sleeves rolled up.

I introduced him to the patients as the real doctor who had come to help me for three weeks. I tried my best to translate the meaning of his degree—Licentiate of the Royal College of Physicians and Surgeons. I think they were impressed, maybe. Anyway they went home that day broadcasting the news, "The real doctor has come to help Dr. Rabbit."

The next day those who were on my waiting list began to come, and you should have seen how that devoted man spent his "vacation." He worked day and night tirelessly serving the multitude that came.

I saw him give a local anesthetic and skillfully correct the young mother's itchy eye. He made an incision on the eyelid below the line of the eyelashes. Then he cut out a section of the skin of the upper eyelid and sewed it up so that it turned the eyelashes out and away from the eye.

The young mother wept with joy, and the waiting multitude ohed and ahed with amazement. I saw him correct the hernia, and again the people ohed and ahed.

I saw him operate on the cataract, and amputate fingers, and mend broken bones. The people ohed and ahed, and still they came.

I saw him examine a poor fellow who had run a splinter of bamboo into his eyeball. The eye was terribly infected, and the proud flesh growing out of the wound looked horrible. Dr. Schilling shook his head and said, "The eyeball will have to come out. There is no possible hope that there is any more sight in it now." I saw him remove that awful-looking eyeball so carefully! So tenderly! And the people ohed and ahed.

Day after day for two weeks he worked. Day and night he worked. The people everywhere talked about it, and the doctor's fame spread wider and wider.

Then one day there came a middle-aged man and an old man with very anxious expressions on their faces. The old man said, "Back at home is a woman—it's my daughter, this man's wife. Her arms and legs are thin as bamboos, but her stomach is as big as a buffalo." I translated the description to Dr. Schilling. He was immediately interested. He asked some very careful, pointed questions, and then he said to me, "Dr. Rabbit, this is evidently one of those rather rare watery cyst cases. If it were cancer, she couldn't have lived seven years with it. These people live only twelve miles away. I have the necessary instruments, and these cases are not usually complicated. It would be a very spectacular operation and would prove a great blessing to God's work. Tell them to come today! I will operate for them."

I translated the doctor's decision. But the men's faces clouded over. "Today?" they gasped.

"Yes, today," said the doctor. "You see, I have only five more days here."

"But not today! We would have to arrange for carriers, and we would have to make sacrifice to the spirits." "Well, tomorrow then," said the doctor. "Bring her tomorrow for sure."

The men turned and ran toward their canoe at the river's edge. "We'll do our best," they called back. But they didn't come tomorrow. Or the next day!

"Dr. Schilling," I said, "they will come about a week after you have gone away. Then what should I do?"

The doctor was only too well acquainted with the jungle way of keeping promises. He looked at me a long minute. Then he said, ''I'll tell you how to drain off some of the fluid. Then you do your best to get her to the surgeon in the Moulmein Hospital. I think he would be glad for one of these cases."

Finally the day of the doctor's departure came. The brass band played and the school choir sang. “Come again next year, Doctor,” I said, and my voice choked.

“I wish I could,” he replied. The motor launch took him off to the river steamer twenty miles away.

Five days after he left, the father and his son-in-law arrived and breathlessly announced, “We’ve got her! We’ve got her! She’s in a house just two and a half miles away, down the river, on the other side.”

“But the doctor has gone away,” I said. “You have come five days too late!”

“Five days too late?” cried the two men together. “We came as quickly as we could. But the spirits! The spirits! It took so long! But now we have their good will. Tell your doctor to come back.”

“The doctor is halfway across the bay to India by this time,” I said. “He can’t come back now.”

“Talk to him on the thunder wire [telegraph],” they cried. “Tell him to come back on the lightning wire.”

“I can talk to him on the thunder wire,” I said, “but the doctor can’t travel back through the lightning wire. The best I can hope for is that he might come next year for another visit.”

The two men looked sadly at each other. They had tried so hard, but they had failed. They were five days too late. At last they looked earnestly into my face and said, “Dr. Rabbit, couldn’t *you* do it?”

I shook my head. “I have neither the skill nor the instruments.”

“Is there nothing you could do?” they persisted.

“I can do a little,” I replied. “I can take away *some* of the fluid.”

I quickly got my things together and with the two men stepped into the motor launch. Very soon we reached the house two and one-half miles down the river where the patient was. The men led me to the house and stood aside while I went up the bamboo ladder. I was about to ask where the patient was when I saw her.

For a moment I was speechless. I felt my eyes bulging; my head was going round and round. I just couldn't believe what I was looking at. The men had described her to Dr. Schilling very accurately. Her arms and legs *were* as thin as bamboos, and her stomach *was* as big as a buffalo, or something else very, very big. When she saw me, she smiled. She thought I was the doctor. At the moment I didn't have the heart to tell her that I wasn't.

I knelt beside her and went quickly to work, and in about an hour I had drained off five gallons and three quarts of fluid! Her face was smiling with happiness. Then I went downstairs to the father and said, "Now, *you* go and tell your daughter that I am not the doctor! Tell her you came five days too late! Tell her I have drained off only some of the fluid and given her temporary relief. In time all that fluid will come back."

"No! No!" said the father. "I couldn't tell her. It would break her heart."

"Then *you* go and tell her," I said to the husband.

"No! No! I couldn't tell her," he cried. "Dr. Rabbit, *you* go and tell her!" So I had to go back upstairs and tell her. She was still smiling as I sat down beside her. The words came hard, but at last I managed to tell her that I was not the doctor. They had come five days too late. I had only been able to give temporary relief. In time the fluid would all come back.

I'm glad you were not there that day. I hope you will never have to see what I saw that morning. As the meaning of my words soaked into her mind, I saw smiling hope slowly crushed from her face, and for the longest minute she looked off into space, seeing nothing. Then she spoke. "You say the doctor might come again next year?"

"He might. I can't say for sure."

"That would be twelve more moons?"

"Yes, twelve more moons."

She looked full into my face and said, "All right, then. All right! You write and tell your doctor! Tell him I'll be lying here on my back counting the moons away till he comes again. I've been lying on my back for seven years. One more year won't be so long."

I went back to my home and sat right down and wrote Dr. Schilling a letter. I told him about the poor woman who would be counting the moons till he came back again. But that night I couldn't sleep. The memory of that smiling hope being slowly crushed from that happy face, and the words, "Counting the moons away till he comes again," haunted me. In the morning I said to my good wife, "You take charge of the mission for a day or two, my dear. I'm going to Moulmein to see if I can find a surgeon to do that operation."

I went, and I did find a surgeon. He was the chief surgeon of the government hospital there. He was interested. He asked many questions, then he said, "Mr. Hare, I'll do the operation on one condition—that you will bring in the patient yourself and stand beside her while I operate, and stay beside her till she wakes up. These country folks are so fearful, it is hard for us to do much for them. But I can see that you have her confidence, and if you are at hand, all will be well."

I went back home rejoicing. I broke the glad news to the patient, her husband, and her father. I agreed to take them all down to Moulmein in the mission launch. "But I can't speak English or Burmese," said the fearful woman.

"I will be with you. I'll do the talking for you," I assured her.

"Oh, yes," she whispered. "But I don't know the way."

"But I know the way," I said. "I know where to go. Remember, I'll be with you. I will not leave you till it is all over."

"Oh, yes!" she whispered. Little by little her fears were calmed. "All right," she said at last. "I won't be afraid if you are with me."

Two days later I stood by the patient in the operating room. "Don't be afraid," I whispered. ''I'm here right near you."

"I won't be afraid if you stay with me," she whispered back.

I saw the doctor drain off three more gallons of fluid. Then I saw him remove a multiple watery cyst. I saw it put on the scales. It weighed forty-nine pounds!

"The biggest I've ever seen," said the surgeon.

They bandaged her up. That is, they bandaged the skin and bones that were left and I sat beside her till she woke up. I saw her eyes flicker. She looked at me and smiled. "Are you still here?" she whispered.

I nodded.

In a few minutes she moved her hands to where the large cyst used to be. A startled look came into her face. "Is it gone?" she gasped.

"Yes. All gone!" I replied.

"And it won't come back?"

"It won't come back."

Then I saw something and heard something that I will remember as long as I live. I saw tears of joy—real tears! Real joy! And I heard her say, “Thank you! Thank you! Thank you!”

Her earnestness brought tears to my eyes. I stepped into the surgeon’s office and described the poor woman’s thankfulness to him. Tears came to his eyes too. Tears of joy.

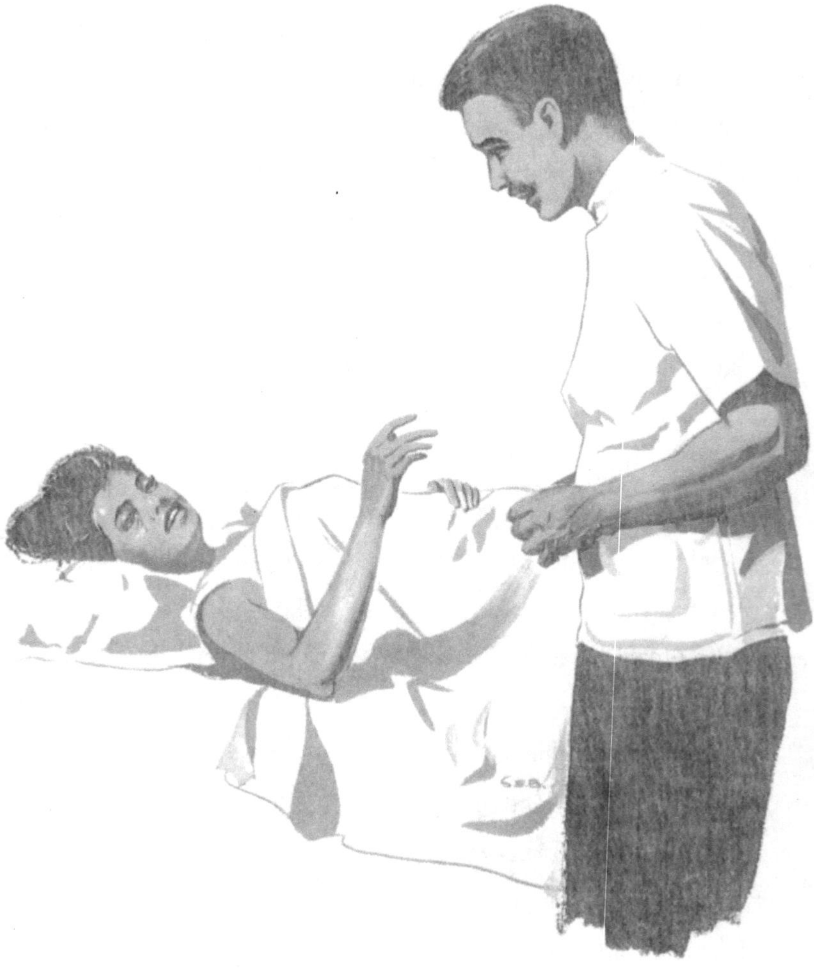

Tears of gratitude filled the patient’s eyes when she saw me standing there and knew the operation was over.

In a month or two she was able to walk around in her village again. And all the people ohed and ahed and cried with joy. I wrote and told Dr. Schilling the good news, and I'm sure a lump came up in his throat and tears of joy came to his eyes as he read of the poor woman's happiness and recalled the strenuous three weeks he had spent with us in our jungle dispensary.

I said to my dear wife, "Mamma Rabbit, this is the life for me! I'd love to stay right here! Why, when we came none of these jungle people believed in God, and now there are three hundred church members. When we came there was only one dispensary; now we have six outstations as well! For a while we worked alone; now we have twenty-two Karens working with us. Oh, I'd love to stay with all these dear needy jungle Karens till Jesus comes."

She said, "I would too."

I said, "We have surely found our own special place; we have surely found real, true happiness here, haven't we?"

And she said, "We surely have."

Good-by Dr. Rabbit and Mamma Rabbit

OUR twenty happy years in our own special mission field had not been without our share of sorrow and sadness. We had one lonely little grave in a cemetery in Rangoon, and one little daughter who had been left deaf, after an attack of spinal meningitis, and now the problem of educating this little deaf girl made it necessary for us to be transferred to California.

For the next seven years, 1934-1941, in cooperation with a splendid lip-reading school in Oakland, we worked hard to teach our little deaf girl to speak. By that time she could speak well enough to go to school with hearing children. So leaving our two older children in Pacific Union College, back we went to our own special place in the Lord's work again, taking our twelve year-old deaf girl and our eight-year-old son, little Peter Rabbit, with us. But we hardly had time to unpack before World War II was upon us, and by July, 1942, we were back in America again. By this time news had come through that our own dear mission station had been burned to the ground, dispensary and all, and that our Karen workers and school students had had to flee to the mountains and the rocks.

It began to look as though we would never get back there again.

But God had other plans. The war ended in 1945, and by the end of 1946 our son Leonard had been graduated from Pacific Union College, was married, and was back in Burma, resurrecting the training school at Myaung Mya. The following year *he moved up to our old mission station and rebuilt it!*

In 1946 I had been appointed to the Sabbath School Department of the General Conference, and in 1954 while conducting a series of Sabbath school workshops in Southern Asia, I had the privilege of spending six days in a workshop in Rangoon!

"Our Dr. Rabbit is coming again," cried our dear Karens in joy. "After twenty years he is coming again!"

After twenty years! Add twenty years to the twenty and thirty-year-old workers, and they would now be the middle-aged responsible ones. Add twenty years to the twelve-to-fifteen-year-old boys and girls, and they would now be the fathers and mothers of a new generation!

So it was, after twenty years I returned to my earlier field of labor. Our former Karen workers from the North and South and East and West had gathered for the workshop in Rangoon. As we met, we wept together with joy. But six days was not long enough to do more than shake hands and ask "Who was who?" Then I was gone again.

Seven more years went by, when in 1961, in harmony with the General Conference policy, Mrs. Hare and I were granted a three-month furlough to Australia. "Dear brethren," I begged, "may we go to Australia via India and Burma and spend two or three weeks in our old mission field?" The brethren said Yes. So we did.

Oh, what a three-week treat that was! We wrote ahead and told

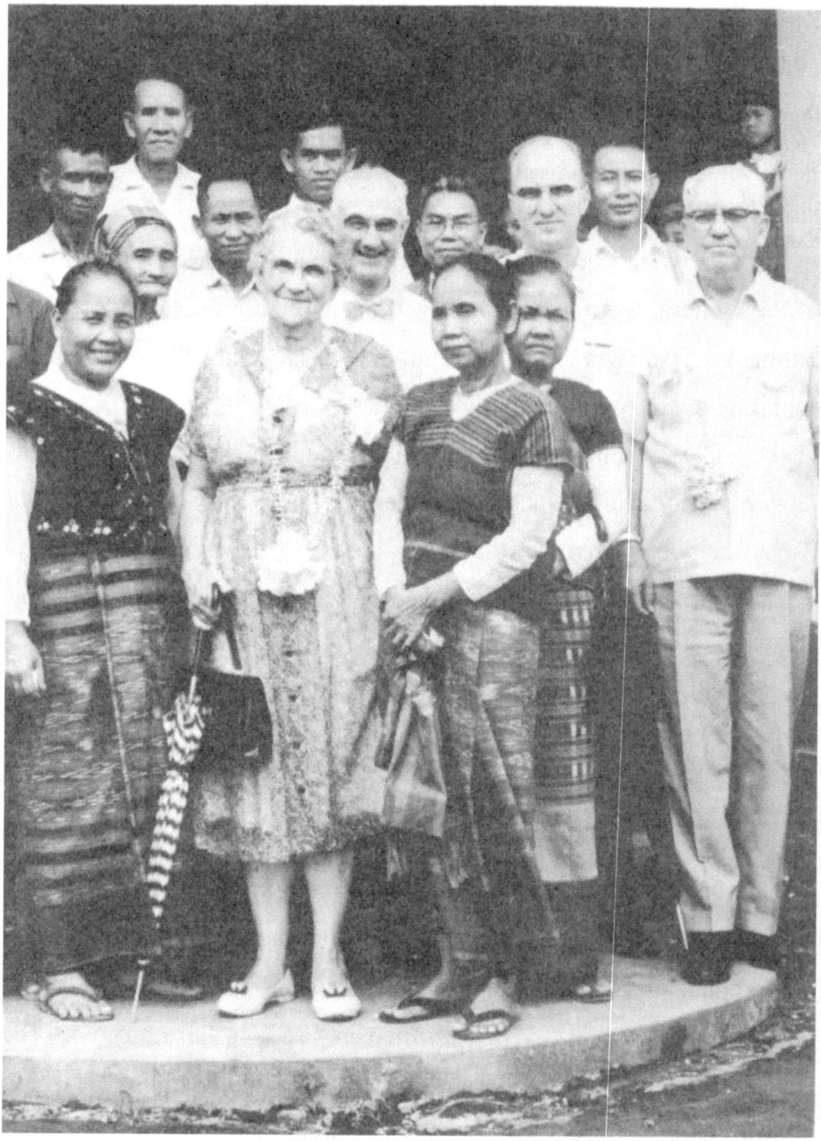

Pastor and Mrs. Eric B. Hare, with their traveling party, receive garlands of welcome on their arrival at Pa-an, Burma.

them we were coming and from village to village it was whispered, "Our dear old Dr. Rabbit and Mamma Rabbit are coming to visit us once more." And on September 13, 1961, we arrived at the airport near Rangoon.As we stepped down from the plane, we noticed a large group of well-dressed people just beyond the customs barrier, carrying flowers and leis. I said to Mrs. Hare, "There must be some V.I.P.'s arriving by this plane also." And we looked around to see if we could make out some government official, some military general, or maybe some movie star. But there was no outstanding personage that we could see. We walked a little nearer, and then we heard them shouting, "Our Dr. Rabbit and Mamma Rabbit have come! They have come!" And all of a sudden we realized that *we* were the V.I.P.'s. We could see at once that Kale Paw, one of our schoolboys who had grown up, was the head of the delegation.

As soon as we had passed customs, the leis were thrown around our necks, and the flowers placed in our hands, and we were nearly smothered with love as fifty or more dear ones crowded forward to shake our hands.

"Dr. Rabbit! Mamma Rabbit! Do you remember me?"

"Mamma Rabbit, look, this is my son!"

"Do you remember that night?"

"Dr. Rabbit, we are grandparents now." And so on, and so on, all the way into the city to our mission headquarters.

"We will give you one more day in Rangoon," said Kale Paw who was the Union Mission secretary at this time, "and then we will fly you over to Paan, where we have relocated your old Ohndaw School. After the war there was too much rebel and bandit action in the vicinity of the Village of Palm Trees so we moved down to

Paan, which is the new government center for the Karen State. For the rest of today and tomorrow we will let you visit with your children here at headquarters and at the hospital."

O what a wonderful two-day visit that was! "Here's K yaw Ba Lay, our head accountant. Do you remember him?"

"Oh, yes, he is Chit Maung's little brother, but I would never recognize him." "And here is Myat Kyaw, the manager of our Bible House."

"Yes."

"And Maung Sein, manager of our printing press."

"Yes, of course. Maung Sein was one of my cornet players in our band." "I still play the cornet!" added Maung Sein with a happy grin.

"And here is Ohn Myit and his good wife, Bu Yin, in the Voice of Prophecy correspondence school. Remember them?"

"Remember? Why I married them!" "And you baptized us too, Dr. Rabbit," added Ohn Myit happily. "I married many others also," I recollected. "Peter and Ma Key."

"Yes, Peter is ordained now and is in charge of our Toungoo church."

"I also married John and Fair One, Hla Baw and Ngwe Sein, Ohn Bwint and Ngwe Shin, Po Kyaw and Sein E, Maung Thein and Yea Mhwe, Maung Kho and Bessie, Tun Maung and Hla Nwe, Tha Kin and Terah."

"Yes, they are all your spiritual children, and tomorrow you will see many of *their* children in our hospital taking the nurse's course."

And on the morrow we certainly did.

“O Mamma, I’m Red Rose, Pink Flower’s daughter.”

“O Mamma, I’m Annie, Yea Mhwe’s little baby girl all grown up, and James, my brother, is taking the nurse’s course too.”

‘’I’m Miriam.”

‘’I’m Moo Tho.”

‘’I’m Ma Pey.”

‘’I’m Paw Gey.”

‘’I’m Hilda.”

‘’I’m TIm Daw. Our mothers and fathers called you Dr. Rabbit and Mamma Rabbit. So you must let us call you Grandpa Rabbit and Grandma Rabbit.” So for this second generation we were Grandpa Rabbit and Grandma Rabbit!

“Here is Kyaw Din, the manager of the hospital.”

“Kyaw Din! I can hardly recognize you.”

“This is Stephen, Thara Peter’s son, the head accountant.”

“Stephen! Do you remember playing motor cars with Lenny when you were little boys?”

“And here’s Pastor Tun Maung, the chaplain of the hospital.”

“Tun Maung! Do you remember when you played the triangle in the band?”

“Indeed I do.”

“And when you were my secretary?”

“Yes, Dr. Rabbit. Those were happy days, and good days to remember. By the way, the nurses are having their junior-senior banquet tonight, and Mamma Rabbit is to be the guest of honor.”

Mamma Rabbit was there. And Mamma Rabbit found it hard to sleep that night when the banquet was over. Her thoughts were too many and too happy. "I can't imagine why these girls should love me so much. They have never seen me before," she whispered.

"But their mothers and fathers more than just saw you, and they have told them plenty," I suggested. "About the way you taught them to sew and cook and keep house, and about the nights when you came—"

"Sh-sh-sh! Don't say any more," said Mamma. "If you say any more I'll cry!"

The next morning we drove to the airport and took a plane to Paan. In forty-five minutes we were there! In our day it would have taken all night and half a day.

Then the greatest thrill of all came Monday morning when they held a farewell service for us. The chapel was crowded. The choir sang. Then Pastor Myat Po, the Karens' silver-tongued orator, president of the Salween Mission, stood up and made his speech. Here is a translation of what he said:

Greetings to Thara and Mamma Hare.

This morning I have the pleasure to have been chosen as the representative of this group, to speak a few words of special welcome to Thara and Mamma.

Most respected Thara, more than forty years ago you planted the first roots of God's work in the Tenasserim district at Ohndaw, the Village of Palm Trees. At first you had only one teacher, Thara Peter, and two school children, Naw Too and Ton Pein. After that each year showed progress. You taught your children many things that have been great blessings to them, such as planting rice, making bricks, digging a well, building homes, singing, the care of the sick, and the playing of band instruments.

In addition to all this you taught us to preach, and you went with us as we conducted village evangelism. As we journeyed you suffered privation with us. You ate the same food. If we had only rice and salt, you ate only rice and salt. When we ate rice and chili paste, you ate rice and chili paste with us. When we ate rice soup, you ate rice soup, and you said, "When my children do not have appetizing food to eat, I could not swallow delicious food all by myself. When there is little to eat, we will all eat the same. When there is a feast, we will all feast together. This will make me happy."

You were not selfish, for you loved others more than you loved yourself. You experienced many privations, but you never complained. You were always happy and rejoiced in the Lord's work. Sometimes we climbed mountains and descended into deep valleys. Sometimes we got lost. We were sometimes hungry and often exhausted but you never showed discouragement. You cheered and encouraged your children; you renewed their strength with songs, so that we were happy all the way. If your children made mistakes, you corrected them in love and with prayer. With reproof you always gave hope. Our greatly respected Thara, although you had to go away, your good example has remained with us and we have tried to do God's work as you did it.

Now if you look at God's work here in Burma, much of it is being carried on by your spiritual children. In the Delta Section, your son Tun Sein is president of the field. In the Chindwin district, your son Baw Dee is in charge. In the Tenasserim Section, your son Myat Po is president of the field. In the south of Burma in the Tavoy district, your son Ohn Bwint, the son of thunder, is the faithful watchman. In the Kayah State, your son Kyaw Din is looking after the work. If you look at our schools, you will find your son Chit Maung principal of the training school at Kyauktaing. In the hospital, your son Tun Maung is the chaplain, and another son is manager. But that is not all. Your son Kalee Paw has become the second king in our Burma Union of Seventh-day Adventists. If you consider all this you have reason to be very proud.

And now our dear mother Mamma Hare. Many years ago you came with our old father and lived in the jungle. Travel was difficult. Food was scarce. Insects and mosquitoes were many. But you suffered them all for us Karens. You are verily a second Mrs. Judson for us Seventh-day Adventist Karens. You helped us in many ways and were always cheerful and kind to us. After you went away your daughters never stopped talking about you. Some said, "When I was born Mamma looked after me like her own child." Another said, "When my breast abscessed and I couldn't feed my child, at night Mamma went without sleep to feed my baby with milk from a bottle." And others said, "Mamma taught me to sew and to cook and to make bread." Ah, yes, they remember and speak of Mamma and the many good things you did for them.

Respected Thara and Mamma, you loved us not only here in Burma but also when you were in America. Our Thara Kale Paw came back from the General Conference in 1958 and told us this. When he went around the world on his way to the conference he went through many countries. Along the way the food was strange and often unpalatable to him, so that he became quite thin.

But when he arrived at Thara and Mamma's house you gave him Burmese food—delicious rice and curry. You gave him a place to sleep and looked after him as your very own son. Because you did this to our representative, it was the same as if you did it to us. Thara Kale Paw came back and told us about the great General Conference, and we listened with delight. He told us of the many churches and camp meetings he visited with you throughout America. He told how you sang Karen songs together, and how you preached together, and we listened with great pleasure. He showed us beautiful pictures that he had taken of former missionaries, great schools, hospitals, beautiful churches, national parks, and great cities. We looked with great pleasure and felt as if we had been in America ourselves.

Wherever Kale Paw goes, and whenever he preaches, he always puts in something about America. So after a while some people said, "Kale Paw is crazy about America." But Thara Kale Paw never stops talking about America. You remember that once Paul preached till midnight in Troas, and one young man, Eutychus, went to sleep and fell out of the window. Well in Konar village Thara Kale Paw preached one Sabbath afternoon from four till nine P.M., and *three* Eutychuscs went to sleep and fell down! We are happy, however, that our representative brought back such a complete report.

Respected Thara and Mamma, if we tried to recall all your goodness to us it would never end. When you are old and retire, may you never forget us and your visit to us at this time. And we will never forget you. We thank God for this privilege of seeing you again. You have worked hard and faithfully among us, and when our dear Saviour comes you will surely hear the words, "Well done, good and faithful servants, you have been faithful over a few things, I will make you ruler over many things. Enter into the joy of thy lord."

And now in closing we say, "May God bless you Thara and Mamma in all of your journey, and may He lengthen your days. Amen. Amen. Amen."

By the time Pastor Myat Po's speech was over Mamma and I were in tears, and so was most of the congregation. When they indicated that they wanted us to speak, I felt helpless. I turned to Mamma Rabbit and whispered, "You go first." She shook her head and said, "No, I can't. You go first."

So I swallowed hard, blew my nose, wiped my eyes, then stood up, and with much difficulty said, "Children and grandchildren, in the Bible we read that God chose a special man for a special work and gave him a special name, Cyrus, one hundred years or more before he was born. In time that special man found his special place and did that special work for God. Even so Mamma Rabbit and I feel that God gave us a special name in order for us to do a special work for Him in a special place."

The congregation murmured pleasantly, "Er—Er."

"And," I continued, "the twenty years we spent with you have been the happiest years of our lives. We thank God for making this visit possible. But we are getting old. Our hair is turning white. We may never see you again on earth. But when we get to heaven, we are going to ask the Lord to let us live again in our own special place, and that place will be with you—our Karen children and grandchildren."

And as I sat down, Mamma Rabbit murmured, "That's what I want to do too!"

Good-by Dr. Rabbit and Mamma Rabbit

www.ingramcontent.com/pod-product-compliance
Lightning Source LLC
LaVergne TN
LVHW101441200926
848483LV00001B/10

* 9 7 8 1 5 7 2 5 8 6 5 1 2 *